FIRST DO NO HARM

A Physician's Burnout and Mental Health Guidebook from Medical School to Retirement

KATHERINE TWOMBLEY, M.D.

Katherine Twombley, M.D.

FIRST DO NO HARM

CONTENTS

Copyright   vii

Acknowledgements   1

FORWARD   **3**

Introduction   5

1 Every Seasoned Physician Was Once a Child: Healing
   from Early Pain   8

2 Medical School and Residency: Surviving the
   Challenges   31

3 Receiving Your Medical License: Out of the Frying
   Pan and into the Fire   60

4 Who Am I? The Identity Crisis   77

5 Burnout and the Missing Off Switch   92

6 Early Career Through Retirement   109

7 Doctors Don't Need to Succumb to the Perfect Storm   134

Conclusion: A Call To Action   156

Bibliography   158

COPYRIGHT

Acknowledgements

I want to thank my family: my daughter (Francesca "Frankie" Chuquimia), my husband (Mohamed Elnemr), my mom (Kay Twombley), my brother (Ashley Twombley) and his family (Carson, Mac, and Will Twombley), and my sister (Tara Twombley) in addition to my many aunts, uncles, and cousins, for allowing me to air some of our family secrets in public. I am so grateful for all of you standing behind me in this project and for seeing the book's potential to help others. I love you all very much!

Besides family, I want to thank some especially dear friends, like Beau Kelly for giving me the support and encouragement to write this book and Justin Bullock for speaking out and not making me feel like I am the only one doing so. You both are amazing people, and I am excited to see what you both do next.

A special shout-out to Scott and Jocelyn Carbonara with Spiritus Communications, for helping me put my thoughts to paper and providing mentorship throughout the writing process. You are both truly gifted.

Thank you to my friends who have been there with me from the beginning. You have stood by my side without judgment and offered nothing except encouragement. I am truly grateful for you.

I really appreciate my Pediatric Nephrology colleagues around the world for walking with me in good times as well as tough times. We are a small but mighty part of medicine, and I am so honored to call you all friends. Thank you for always being there for me.

Finally, I want to thank my father (a.k.a., my hero) who inspired me to be the person I am today. I love you and miss you more than you will ever know.

Forward

First Do No Harm:
A Physician's Burnout and Mental Health Survival Guide
from Medical School to Retirement

As a specialist in physician health, I am honored to write the Foreword for Dr Twombley's unique and important book. She is highly qualified – an accomplished academic pediatric nephrologist, a sought-after lecturer in physician burnout and wellness, and tragically, the daughter of a beloved country doctor who took his life August 17, 2011. The lived experience of those who have lost a loved one to suicide is distinctive and gives this book an experiential, heartfelt context that permeates every page. This sets it apart alongside the many fine publications addressing burnout and surviving in today's medical world.

We are introduced to the author's father James Michael Twombley, MD at the outset and learn a bit about him as a father, family man, dedicated physician, a man of values and principles, including compassion and generosity. She then takes the reader on a developmental path beginning with the childhood of physicians, too often neglected in our understanding of the humanness of doctors, including our vulnerabilities. Her review of early childhood trauma and its impact, and Adverse Childhood Experiences, is scholarly and buttressed with insights from psychology, philosophy, and literature. Dr Twombley continues this pattern as she moves through medical training, graduating and licensure, early career, burnout, mid to late career, and retirement. She speaks directly to the reader with sage advice based on her own personal experience in medicine, her father's, and physician health researchers and authors.

Dr Twombley pulls no punches as she, later in the book, dissects her father's workaholism, struggles with intimacy, tendency to withdraw to his "man's cave", deteriorating mental health, drinking and smoking, tinkering with his gun collection, faltering work performance, and the specifics of his suicide. The book ends with a Call to Action, a collective outreach to physicians and the medical world at large. We must come together and fight the systemic forces and paralyzing stigma that are making doctors sick and putting them at risk of suicide.

The last line of her magnificent book is precious, a loving paean to her father: "If I can prevent one physician death from telling his story, then it is worth every single tear I have shed while writing it." *First Do No Harm* is an extremely useful resource for medical students and physicians, their families, their teachers and those who treat them.

Michael F Myers, MD
Professor of Clinical Psychiatry
SUNY Downstate Health Sciences University
Brooklyn, NY
And author "Why Physicians Die by Suicide: Lessons Learned from Their Families and Others Who Cared"

Introduction

My father, James Michael Twombley, MD, (a.k.a., Mike) inspired me to follow him into medicine, where I now serve as a pediatric nephrologist. I watched him serve for several decades as a loving and highly respected country doctor with an unforgettable bedside manner. All who knew him were awed by his knowledge as well as his compassion, wit, and generosity. Doctor T—as his patients, colleagues, and even his loving family called him—never let a patient's inability to pay stop him from providing the best level of care, even if it meant paying out of his own pocket.

My dad was a great father too. He and my mother raised us with a strong sense of responsibility and what one might call "high morals." To demonstrate this, my family attended church every time the doors were open. We never had alcohol in our house. Instead of leaving us so they could attend parties, concerts, movies, or other social events, my parents stayed home with us when we were children. We knew that we were their priority.

Daddy also taught me how to respect wildlife and not be afraid of frogs, lizards, and snakes. He kept me entertained by showing me how to get a lizard to bite my ears so that they looked like earrings, and how to build homemade cherry bombs out of cat food tins. He once took me on a daddy-daughter trip to Disney World where I had his undivided attention each night at the park.

Growing up, I never doubted how much he loved us. In fact, he had so much love in his heart that after a short time as empty nesters, my mom and dad adopted my sister so they could share their abundance of love with her too.

Given all the cherished memories I have of my father, his death by suicide on August 17, 2011, sent me reeling.

I have spent the decade-plus since searching for answers that are undoubtedly impossible to find. As a physician myself, I wondered what I might have missed that led my dad to that last act of despair. *Had there been signs? What could I have done to intervene?* And to address the bigger picture, I asked myself, *Why are doctors "burning out," suffering in silence, and taking their own lives? Am I, too, at risk of taking my life like my father did? As physicians, and as a society, is there anything we can do to reverse this trend?*

After years of not having definitive answers about my father's mental health or his decision to end his life, I decided that the best way to honor his memory was to do whatever I could to educate others on the rarely discussed truths about physician mental health and suicide. After exploring the topic, I've now decided to share my findings in this book. I wrote this book for those—

- Considering the field of medicine,
- Enrolled in medical school,
- Practicing medicine,
- Loving someone in the medical field, or
- Seeking to better understand physician mental health (including suicide) or help someone who may be struggling; this may be a psychologist/therapist, healthcare leader, or colleague of physicians.

In *First Do No Harm: A Physician's Burnout and Mental Health Survival Guide from Medical School to Retirement,* I'll share parts of my father's life to highlight potential events that contributed to his death. Additionally, for those of you who are medical providers, I will make recommendations to help you safeguard your mental *and* physical health as you practice. Finally, I'll offer insights for those who love someone working in the medical field, so you can look for potential warning signs.

As you read, you may see yourself in some of these situations or recognize traits of someone you know or love. Or you may be reading this because you're entering medical school or considering a role in medicine, and you want to know the ins and outs of protecting your mental health before it becomes a crisis. My hope is that any connections you make to the book's content will help you seek guidance or assist others in finding healing.

—Katherine E. Twombley, M.D.

Every Seasoned Physician Was Once a Child: Healing from Early Pain

ER, Grey's Anatomy, General Hospital, The Good Doctor, Chicago Med, and other televisions dramas might offer binge-worthy entertainment, but they don't closely compare to the real healthcare field. Sure, the characters wear the same uniforms and use the same medical terminology, but the on-screen drama is just as often due to their steamy extramarital affairs as with their grappling with life-and-death decisions. Actual medical doctors, however, must balance pressures including their patients' sometimes precarious well-being, compliance regulations, health insurance stipulations, scheduling and staffing pressures—along with interpersonal dynamics inherent in any workplace. And that's just a start to the long list of factors that might keep doctors up at night.

While it would be easy to view working in healthcare as a battle of doctor versus disease, as you can surmise from this list, the biggest challenge facing doctors is simply overwhelming *stress*. Medical doctors are human beings too, and as such, they struggle with many of the same issues that people in other fields face—while also facing pressures that are unique to the field. We will explore these factors in this book.

So, what makes a doctor, and why enter the field? The average person recognizes that doctors need a combination of intelligence and determination to complete medical school. Then, after years of schooling and training, doctors get paid well for their skills. In fact, of the twenty-five top paying jobs in the US, only three careers (chief executives, aviators, and information technology managers) come from outside healthcare (Probasco 2023).

Some might conclude that smart, determined, and financially well-off people have every advantage in life. But they would be wrong. Healthcare professionals face very real yet often hidden stressors, as stated. The 2019 year-end edition of the *Medical Economics Journal* describes these stressors in more detail, as they wrote a list of the top ten challenges that physicians would face in the coming year (Medical Economics 2019, 6-19). Here are the most relevant ones you should know:

- **Administrative burdens.** Think of the myriad tasks that keep doctors from treating patients. Tasks like intervening to get insurance to pay for important procedures or medications or ensuring that visits are properly documented in patients' charts, takes physicians away from direct care. It's necessary work, but those tasks are often viewed as the least rewarding. Many doctors felt compelled to join healthcare to heal or help patients, but the reality is they must spend significant time jumping through administrative hoops.

- **Getting paid.** Providing services doesn't always mean getting compensated. Why? Doctors must complete reams of increasingly complex, ever-changing forms linked to quality metrics, patient outcomes, coding, and more tasks just to get paid for their work.

- **Increased healthcare competition.** Few practices are the "only game in town." Competition means clinics and hospitals must offer extended hours, conveniences, and access channels. In practical terms, competition often forces healthcare workers (HCWs) to work longer hours just to stay in business. And for many doctors, pressure comes from their leaders who must continually strive to differentiate their practice, often reporting to a board of directors who expect results.
- **Avoiding lawsuits.** Doctors work in a field where every action can have an adverse impact on the health of another person, up to and including death. Lawsuits are far from rare, and few people work best when someone is looking over their shoulders and second-guessing their every decision.
- **Getting Promoted.** Medical doctors who work in academia start at the bottom of the totem pole. To get promoted, they must publish articles, receive national recognition, give talks at meetings, be awarded grants, and teach. Some institutions give them a set time frame to get promoted to the next level. These are called "up or out" institutions because they can either move up, or they need to move out.

Of course, that article came out before most of the world ever heard of COVID-19. Since the pandemic, healthcare workers have experienced even greater stress. The National Institute of Health (NIH) published an article that spotlights how COVID-19 unleashed severe impacts on the health and well-being of HCWs (Gupta et al. 2021, 282-284):

1. Increased psychological stress and anxiety
2. High rate of infection and death

3. Reduced sleep health
4. Increased drug use
5. Burnout
6. Increased financial hardship
7. Suicidal ideation
8. Suicide

Even years into the pandemic, many practices and healthcare systems struggled to remain fully staffed. Some HCWs quit during the pandemic out of fear of bringing COVID home to their families; others left when their facilities mandated each HCW receive a COVID vaccine. Staff shortages put more work on the doctors and HCWs remaining. In other words, doctors had plenty of stressors prior to COVID, and the pandemic exacerbated the existing issues.

My Father: A Case of Unresolved Childhood Trauma

Imagine a physician or other healthcare worker bringing untreated childhood trauma to their job. Their role is stressful on a good day. COVID-19 made the work exponentially more stressful. When that additional weight is dropped on top of a foundation already damaged from childhood trauma, it can create disastrous results.

Physicians weren't born with MDs. They started off as children, just like everyone else. The kind of childhood they experienced had a great impact on the kind of adult—and doctor—they became. For that reason, it's worth exploring how childhood trauma can lead to dysfunction in a physician's adult life.

My father is a prime example of this. He rarely talked about his early life, but from what little he shared—along with interviews I conducted after he passed—I know he had an unhappy childhood. Unresolved childhood trauma then followed him throughout his entire life. No matter what he accomplished (he was an Eagle Scout, the first in his family to go to medical school, Medical Director of Emergency Medical Services in Dillon County, Medical Director of the Emergency Department at Saint Eugene Community Hospital/ McLeod Dillon, Physician of the Year in1984, President of the South Carolina Rheumatism Society, and other distinctions), the pain from his childhood went with him. He could earn degrees, awards, and public accolades, but he never confronted the demons of his past.

Born during the marriage of Glen Gregory and Louise Belle, Mike entered the world on July 30, 1946. A couple of years later, his sister, Linda, joined the family. But the marriage between Louise and Glen wouldn't last.

Glen had always wanted to serve in the military, so he lied about his age to enter the US Army before he reached the legal age of enlistment. He ended up a decorated war hero and a raging alcoholic. After the war, he worked for the government in Maryland. One day while returning home from work, he stopped to fix a flat tire on his car. While he changed the tire, he got hit by another car. His injuries were so extensive that the doctors told him he would never walk again.

Equally damaging to their marriage was Louise's secretive and demanding personality. After my father's death, I learned that Louise worked for the Office of Strategic Services (OSS), a federal intelligence agency responsible for collecting and analyzing strategic information, disseminating propaganda, creating subversion, and, eventually, planning post-war activities. Shortly after World War II, the OSS became the Central Intelligence Agency (CIA). While I have no idea what Louise did for the spy agency, I learned that she frequently travelled across the country for work.

Whatever her role, Louise must have been well-connected within the agency. Shortly after Linda was born, Louise asked Glen for a divorce. She also asked him to surrender his parental rights to both Mike and Linda. Believing he was permanently disabled, Glen agreed so that his children could have a better life. Louise then married William R. Twombley, who she was already pregnant by, and the two had a baby named Lisa. Twombley adopted Mike and Linda. Without talking to Mike and Linda about her divorce or new husband, Louise simply told the children that their new last name was Twombley.

My mother told me that Dad admitted to her that this was one of the most devastating times in his life. Given no explanation or time to process or even say goodbye to his father, eight-year-old Mike started to lose his identity. And to make things even worse for Mike, all of this happened in the 1940s when divorce was considered taboo.

Louise didn't stay married to Twombley. I can't find a divorce certificate for them, but I learned why that is. Since Louise worked for the OSS/CIA, she was able to pull some strings. She had my father's adoption—and we think her divorce records to Twombley —sealed with a one-hundred-year classification on them that started sometime in the late 1940s to early 1950s. My mother told me that my father tried to unlock those records but learned it would take an act of God to unseal them. Louise also used her connections within the government to keep Dad out of the Vietnam War after he was drafted. As the highest-ranking OSS/CIA civilian at Shaw Airforce base in Sumpter, SC at that time (or so we have been told), Louise was able to keep her son out of military service and to keep her personal life a secret.

By all accounts, my Grandma Louise hated my Grandpa Glen Gregory. I've never heard the reason why she held so much bitterness towards this man. I met Glen when I was in high school. He readily admitted that he had returned from the war an alcoholic who, by the way, learned to walk again. He seemed like a very kind human being. But I noticed one more thing: Dad looked like a carbon copy of Glen.

My father thought Louise remained cold to him because of his resemblance to his father, Glen. I can verify that Dad seemed like a pariah at our annual dinners at Grandma Louise's house. Grandma built strong relationships with Linda and Lisa as well as their children. My cousins even spent summers with Louise, and they always spoke lovingly of her. The experiences my brother and I had with Grandma Louise were completely different. She scared me. While she wasn't overtly mean, she threw off a kind of aura that made me fear her. No affection, no kind words. To us, Grandma Louise was just an older woman who we obligingly visited once a year for Thanksgiving.

Dad grew up in a house where his mother travelled regularly for work, and he was either dropped off at relatives' homes or left alone when she left town. While he made excellent grades in school, I believe he would have also scored high on the Adverse Childhood Experiences (ACE) test, which isn't a good thing. The ACE is a ten-question questionnaire that evaluates the level of abuse, neglect, and household challenges that occurred in one's childhood from ages zero to seventeen years (see later in this chapter for the specific questions).

My father entered a world without security or parental attachment by the time he reached eight years of age. When his biological father relinquished his parenting rights before a man named Twombley entered his family's home, adopted him and his sister, changed their last name, gave them a half-sister, and then left without saying goodbye, my dad was impacted in ways that would follow him into adulthood.

Time, on its own, doesn't erase the damage from childhood trauma. The impact doesn't disappear once that child enters adolescence and adulthood. When a traumatized child reaches sixty years old, unless they have sought intervention, they are a traumatized adult in an older body. No advanced degrees, prestige, or money heals those wounds.

Adults who have lived through childhood trauma can recover and heal, but it requires work. Left unresolved, the effect of childhood trauma increases over time.

The Life-Long Impact of Unresolved Childhood Trauma: Seven Consequences

Children growing up with trauma develop coping skills to manage circumstances they can't control or change. While those skills allow them to survive childhood, different skills are required to be successful adults, as they hopefully navigate into a world without such trauma.

The National Child Traumatic Stress Network summarizes the most common struggles adults living with unresolved childhood trauma experience. Let's explore seven consequences.

1. Poor Attachment and Relationships Adult children of trauma learn that they are on their own, since no one in their lives cares enough about them to help. As a result, they view themselves and the world as a bad, unsafe place. They struggle to form strong, healthy relationships, and they are slow to trust others. Their internal monologue echoes the message, *I can't rely on anyone but myself.*

2. Recurring Physical and Mental Struggles Adult children of trauma often live with a low stress threshold. Even when facing low to moderate amounts of stress, they may show signs of physiological reactivity, like increased breathing or pulse. Some over- or under-react in response to perceived stress, and they may partake in risky behaviors such as smoking, substance abuse, poor diet, high-risk sex, reckless driving, and so on. They may feel, *Life is too much; I must find ways to escape this overwhelming pressure.*

3. Difficulty Identifying, Sharing, and Managing Emotions Adult children of trauma may struggle to read the emotions of others. But they're just as likely to fail in understanding, processing, and responding to their own emotions. At times, they can be unpredictable and explosive, and they often have difficulty calming themselves down. This can lead to instability in their relationships. They are also more prone to suffer from depression, anxiety, and anger than those who didn't experience childhood trauma. They may ask themselves, *Why doesn't anyone understand me?* While also thinking, *Why does this keep happening to me?*

4. Dissociation Adult children of trauma can dissociate, or "check out," when they feel emotionally triggered. As children, they learned to detach from stressful situations and people by stepping outside of themselves to enter a "safer" place. Some seem to daydream, while others may perceive that they've left their bodies as they observe their lives from a safe distance. Most often, dissociating adults don't seem fully present in the moment. They may unconsciously sense, *Anywhere is better than here.*

5. Inability to Self-Regulate Behavior Adult children of trauma often have low impulse control and act without thinking through all the consequences of their behavior. For my dad, that meant playing practical jokes in college, and as an adult, that often led to him getting disciplined or receiving unintended consequences. This trait can lead to shameful thoughts like, *I can't believe I did that again—making a fool of myself. Why can't I stop?*

6. *Cognitive Challenges* Adult children of trauma often *react* instead of *responding* to challenges due to their failure to plan and accurately anticipate the consequences of their actions. They may feel, *This is a threat, and I must beat it back immediately.* Or they may realize, *I can't believe I did that again. When will I use my head?*

7. *Lack of Hope* Adult children of trauma didn't receive nurturing, guidance, and protection from their caregivers, causing them to develop a distorted sense of self-worth and value. Many suffer with shame, guilt, low self-esteem, and a poor self-image. As a result, they view their lives as purposeless, the world as meaningless, and their power to effect positive change as futile (Peterson 2018). They may conclude, *Why bother? I'll mess up anyway, or someone won't give me the credit I deserve.*

Children have no expectations about what to expect from life except their own experiences. Whatever happens in childhood imprints on how that child views the world, builds relationships, cares for themselves, and plans their futures. If you enjoyed a happy, carefree childhood, those early experiences remain with you. If you had a traumatic childhood, those early experiences remain with you—unless you confront them and heal from them.

Addressing Childhood Trauma as a Physician: How to Begin Healing

Adult victims of childhood trauma can heal and live happy, productive, and successful lives, but it doesn't happen automatically.

Doctors-in-training participate in clinical rotations, also known as clerkships. During this time, residents work for several weeks in various medical disciplines under the direction of an experienced physician. One of the disciplines residents work in is psychiatry and behavioral health.

Does the time completing a psychiatry rotation make doctors experts in emotional trauma? Absolutely not. Clinical rotations give doctors just a small taste of diagnosing and treating patients to see if this is the field the student would be interested in pursuing as a career. A psychiatric rotation alone doesn't equip doctors to resolve their own struggles or work through their own childhood trauma. Before a doctor can gain board certification in an area such as psychiatry and truly be versed in the field, they must go through four additional years of training after earning their doctor of medicine (MD) degree; and that still doesn't mean they've dealt with their own traumas.

So how does this affect physicians-in-training? Imagine going through childhood trauma and having the previously listed challenges as a medical student. Victims of childhood trauma often live in or reflect on the past where they replay past episodes of abuse or neglect. And past events serve as a lens for how victims view the present and plan for the future. How do you think a medical student with a happy and healthy childhood—versus a physician with unresolved childhood trauma—would react to seeing an abuse victim during an emergency medicine rotation, a sexual assault victim on a gynecology rotation, a child abuse victim on a pediatric rotation, or an alcoholic on a psychiatric rotation?

Once those medical students become physicians, the trauma reminders can continue. For example, doctors working in emergency departments (EDs) will treat a vast range of traumas: rape, sexual abuse, sexual assault, domestic violence, car accidents, and violent assault. Is it any surprise that doctors who have had personal traumas such as these can find treating these patients triggering? A doctor with unresolved trauma or post-traumatic stress disorder (PTSD) may experience a rush of triggering emotions that inhibits the executive function of their brains (Aupperle et al. 2012, 686-94). Consider these ED scenarios:

- The doctor who was sexually assaulted as a child treating a rape victim;
- The doctor whose father died by suicide fighting to save someone who attempted suicide; or
- The doctor whose mother died in a car accident treating a whole family severely wounded after a freeway pileup.

Even medical specialties outside of the ED aren't free of potential trauma triggers. Consider:

- The psychiatrist who witnessed verbal and physical abuse as a child providing marital counseling to a severely abusive spouse;
- The family practitioner who lost a parent to cancer palpating an abdomen and discovering a suspicious lesion; or
- The pediatrician who lost a young sibling to a rare disease recognizing the symptoms of the same disease in an infant patient.

Any clinician facing a patient with trauma can become triggered, but those who have had similar traumas might not be capable of making the best decisions for their patients. Revisit the seven consequences of childhood trauma to imagine how these triggers can affect physicians in the moment of caregiving—and later when they get home. Reacting instead of responding to a medical emergency, for example, could mean the difference between life and death. While the consequence to patients isn't typically this severe, there's a large, grayer area where distraction, depression, and deteriorating mental and physical health can take a toll on outcomes—both to the physician and patient they are serving. And this toll can be cumulative.

Considering the potential negative outcomes in these scenarios, anyone interested in serving as a healthcare professional owes it to themselves, their loved ones, and their patients to evaluate their childhood experiences for trauma. So what can you do about it?

Evaluate Your Adverse Childhood Experiences (ACEs)

This may all sound depressing and defeating so far, and it certainly is alarming. If you experienced childhood trauma (or find yourself wondering if you did), however, it doesn't mean you're heading for a cliff with no steering wheel to maneuver you out of harm's way. There is hope, and there are solutions. Healing so that you can thrive in your practice—and your life—is possible awareness of your vulnerabilities. And a good place to start is with exploration of your ACEs, as mentioned earlier.

In the mid-1990s, the Centers for Disease Control and Kaiser Permanente launched its initial Adverse Childhood Experience (ACE) study to determine the extent that early childhood trauma impacts adults later in life. The original study focused on three categories: abuse, household challenges, and neglect.

The ACE questionnaire has ten questions. Read the following questions and give yourself one point for each "yes" answer. When you're done, total the points to arrive at your cumulative number of ACEs.

Before your eighteenth birthday:

1. Did a parent or other adult in the household often or very often...

   • Swear at you, insult you, put you down, or humiliate you? or

- Act in a way that made you afraid that you might be physically hurt?

2. Did a parent or other adult in the household often or very often...

- Push, grab, slap, or throw something at you? or
- Ever hit you so hard that you had marks or were injured?

3. Did an adult or person at least five years older than you ever...

- Touch or fondle you or have you touch their body in a sexual way? or
- Attempt or actually have oral, anal, or vaginal intercourse with you?

4. Did you often or very often feel that...

- No one in your family loved you or thought you were important or special? or
- Your family didn't look out for each other, feel close to each other, or support each other?

5. Did you often or very often feel that...

- You didn't have enough to eat, had to wear dirty clothes, and had no one to protect you? or
- Your parents were too drunk or high to take care of you or take you to the doctor if you needed it?

6. Were your parents ever separated or divorced?

- Was your mother or stepmother:
  Often or very often pushed, grabbed, slapped, or had something thrown at her? or
- Sometimes, often, or very often kicked, bitten, hit with a fist, or hit with something hard?

7. Ever repeatedly hit over at least a few minutes or threatened with a gun or knife?

8. Did you live with anyone who was a problem drinker or alcoholic, or who used street drugs?

9. Was a household member depressed or mentally ill, or did a household member attempt suicide?

10. Did a household member go to prison?

The higher the number, the greater the risk for a person to carry emotional and behavioral damage into adulthood (Starecheski 2015). An ACE score of 3 or more is considered high. My father had a score of at least 4.

More specifically, according to research, those who score highest on the ACE are prone to suffer the following consequences as adults (Rymanowicz 2018):

- Risky health behaviors
- Chronic health conditions
- Low life potential
- Early death

Another source suggests that signs of childhood trauma in adults show up in four common ways (Roncero 2021):

1. Difficulty establishing healthy relationships
2. Hyper-vigilance (feeling threatened or on high-alert)

3. Depression and anxiety
4. Post-traumatic stress disorder (PTSD)

Jamie lost her father when she was eleven years old. Her mother immediately started dating and traveling out-of-state to be with her new boyfriend, leaving Jamie at home for weeks at a time with her teenage sister. Jamie's sister regularly stayed with friends, leaving the eleven-year-old girl home alone.

Jamie didn't know how to start a fire in the wood stove, the only heat source for the home. More than once she woke up and found the water in the dog dish next to the stove frozen over. With neither heat nor food in her house, Jamie suffered in silence.

Jamie's mother eventually returned home with her new boyfriend who sexually and physically abused Jamie and then threatened to send her away if she told anyone. Terrified and violated, Jamie determined to be neither seen nor heard in her home for the next several years.

A few years passed. Jamie's mother broke up with her abusive boyfriend and met a nice man. The two married and made a good home for Jamie. But the damage had been done. Jamie grew to distrust others. Never having dealt with the death of her biological father, Jamie started believing that she, too, would die young and quickly. She began drinking, taking drugs, shoplifting, and making other poor choices. Pregnant, she dropped out of high school in her senior year, moved in with her boyfriend, and joined him on a drive that took a felonious turn when he committed an armed robbery in which she became his unwitting accomplice and received jail time.

From age eleven through eighteen, Jamie lived through several adverse childhood experiences that she replayed in her mind into adulthood. After a suicide attempt, Jamie was involuntarily committed to a psychiatric care facility where she entered counseling for the first time in her life.

Get Help

Children who grew up in an environment of rejection, criticism, and abandonment often become their own worst critics. They blame themselves for whatever happens—except for positive events. When something good happens, they view happy circumstances as if they never happened. Instead of rejoicing at positive events, they respond to them with fear and trepidation, as if they're waiting for the other shoe to drop. Others, like my father, don't feel worthy of the praise when they do something good.

Researchers found that 15 to 43 percent of children experience at least one significant trauma (US Dept. of Veterans Affairs 2018). Several of those children will develop post traumatic stress disorder (PTSD).

You can overcome past traumas with the right help. Behavioral health treatment has come light years from the days of trepanation (drilling holes in someone's skull to release evil spirits), lobotomies, and insulin coma therapies. While psychotherapists can use countless methodologies to guide clients through trauma, the following three techniques are most popular for addressing PTSD and childhood trauma.

Not everyone suffering from mental health challenges had traumatic childhoods. Some struggling with mental health issues had idyllic childhoods, yet they still suffer from chemical imbalances that can cause depression, anxiety, bipolar disorder, and other conditions.

Being diagnosed with a mental health condition early in life can have advantages. First, an early diagnosis can put a treatment plan in place that may involve medication and counseling. Second, it can help a person with mental health struggles create and tap into a safety plan and deep support network. Finally, any treatment plan applied and followed before attending college or medical school means the student will have experience in getting needed support before the stress of schooling increases.

But keep this in mind: *having* a treatment plan isn't the same as *applying* a treatment plan. An unfollowed plan of action yields the same results as having no plan. So if you've been prescribed medication and counseling, it's critical that you follow the plan and keep your support network close.

Cognitive Behavioral Therapy (CBT). Those who suffer childhood trauma learn coping mechanisms to help them survive in a world where they feel threatened. Over time, those coping mechanisms become habits, or patterns of behavior. When someone with trauma encounters a potentially threatening event, they get triggered, leading them to negative thoughts, emotions, behavior, and physical responses.

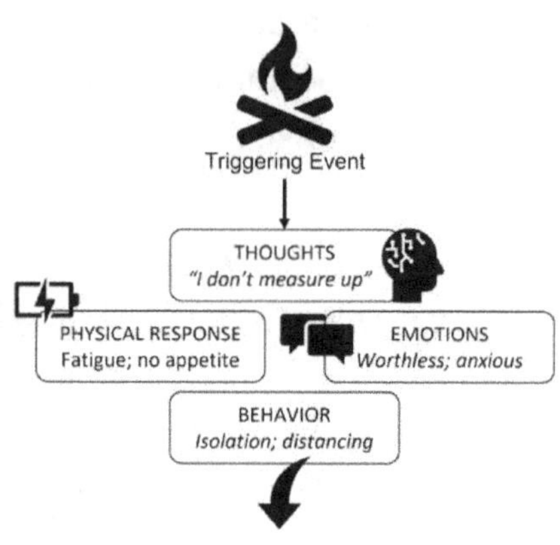

CBT helps people understand how their behaviors are driven by their thoughts and feelings. This method of therapy empowers people to change their thoughts and feelings, recognize the genesis of their behavioral patterns, and create new, healthy patterns. It thereby enables those who have experienced trauma to uncouple threatening events and break the negative pattern that follows.

Narrative Exposure Therapy (NET). Psychologists created the term *negativity bias* to describe the human tendency to feel the consequences of negative experiences more than positive ones. When test subjects are asked to recall memorable events from childhood, they have an easier time recalling negative experiences than positive ones. Therapists use NET to guide clients through the process of examining their life stories. Initially, the client's narrative focuses on traumatic events. Eventually, the therapist helps a client reconstruct the many positive events that coexisted with the trauma. This process helps people view their lives as a whole—with both positive and negative experiences—instead of as one that is terribly lobsided and rooted only in trauma.

Eye Movement Desensitization and Reprocessing (EMDR). EMDR therapy reduces the negative emotions attached to traumatic events. EMDR focuses on traumatic memories people hold, but it also uses bilateral stimulation that can include eye movement, tapping, sounds, or vibrations. By adding bilateral stimulation while retelling and reliving traumatic events, the client can create distance from, and new emotional connections to, painful memories.

According to the EMDR Institute, clients sift through PTSD and childhood traumas using their own accelerated intellectual and emotional processes. After a few sessions, most clients feel empowered by the very experiences that once traumatized them (EMDR 2020). Instead of feeling shame or anger for past traumas, clients teach themselves to say triumphantly, "I lived through hell, but I'm stronger because of it!"

Name It to Tame It

Beyond knowing that you have lived through childhood trauma, practice what psychiatrist Daniel Siegel refers to as "name it to tame it" (Mindful Staff 2020). I find this skill particularly helpful.

Adults who were traumatized as children often live in the past, continually reliving times of high stress and trauma even in the absence of actual threats, as described in the examples of medical doctors in triggering situations. When confronted with painful memories, these adults reengage in the same fight/flight/freeze coping mechanisms they used when they were children, and their memories reignite strong negative emotions.

Here's an example of what it looks like when the past plays out in the present:

1. A current event reminds you of a past trauma.
2. Your body responds just like it did during your past trauma (with increased heart rate and breathing).
3. You tell yourself, "Here we go again!"
4. You reexperience the feelings you had during past trauma (fear, anger, hurt, rejection, humiliation, etc.).
5. You try to deny your negative emotions and work through them
6. Your body, under the additional stress from denying your negative emotions, becomes more tense and releases more stress hormones.
7. You act out physically or with an emotional outburst.

As you can imagine, this behavior would not take you far in medical school or your medical practice—or in your personal life. Instead of letting past traumas hijack your current emotions in this way—potentially derailing your career—you can name your emotion as you experience it. By practicing *name it to tame it*, you can change your pattern of dealing with present stresses caused from past traumas. The process looks like this:

1. A current event reminds you of a past trauma.
2. Your body responds like it did during your past trauma.
3. You acknowledge that this situation bothers you, and you exhale slowly.
4. You label the emotion you are feeling (such as fear).
5. You tell yourself, "I am afraid, but I am also safe" while breathing in slowly.

6. You repeat to yourself, "I am afraid, but I am also safe" while continuing to breath in slowly and breath out even more slowly.
7. Your heart rate and breathing slow down until you can *respond* to the actual event instead of *reacting* to your negative emotions.

Changing these patterns begins with awareness that the threat in front of you isn't real (if it's not a new, actual threat like another abuse). The situation that reminds you of the past, even if unconsciously, is *not* the same. You're an adult now, not a child with no options, and you can make adult decisions. You can steer yourself to safety or reassure yourself that you're already safe.

But it's easy to revert to the same reaction unless you become aware of it and choose to change it.

Think of a tractor that creates ruts in the mud after a storm. Those ruts dry when the sun comes out, but the tractor still fall into the ruts. It takes intention to steer clear of the ruts and carve a new path.

Next time you find your body tensing up in response to a trigger, pause, breathe, and ask yourself if your reaction is appropriate to the threat in front of you. If it's not, practice the seven steps listed, and carve a new route to your intended emotion.

Chapter 1 Summary

Trauma experienced in childhood follows us throughout our entire lives. Unless we choose to confront and heal from our traumas, we will follow the habits, patterns, and coping mechanisms developed in childhood to deal with situations that trigger and threaten us.

Doctors are not immune from ACEs. And doctors with childhood trauma are more likely to become triggered when treating patients who have experienced similar traumas. In fact, very few people entering medical school come from a background of privilege or even from a family or doctors. Given the additional stress doctors face in training and on the job, it's even more imperative for them to deal with past traumatic experiences; otherwise, they may become a risk to themselves and their patients.

Experiencing childhood trauma is but one potential challenge that doctors face, and I hope you feel encouraged by knowing some of the tools that exist to overcome it. In the next chapter, I'll explain how schooling and training pile even greater stress on healthcare professionals—and what you can do about it.

Medical School and Residency: Surviving the Challenges

When you're a child, you create a picture of what your adult life will entail. You might develop an altruistic vision of serving people across the world or solving a global crisis. Or perhaps you imagine doing all the long-forbidden things, like jumping on the bed and eating Cap'n Crunch cereal straight from the box.

A child trying to imagine what it's like to be a doctor may initially rely on television and movies that depict the role. As the child grows into a teen and does their own research, they may assume that becoming a doctor is about learning about thousands of medications and diseases, passing medical school, making accurate diagnoses, and prescribing the right medication. When entering the field of medicine, however, those won't constitute all the tasks, or even the ones that are the most challenging. Even when doctors complete rotations in medical school, they still don't have the full picture of what it's like to be a doctor.

Being a doctor means fighting for everything a patient needs— which includes navigating complex documentation and health insurance stipulations. Yet this isn't taught in medical school. Students don't learn how to complete the hundreds of various forms required so their patients can get the necessary tests. There's no class on what documentation and codes each insurance provider needs before they will reimburse for the treatment. And medical students aren't taught what the patients will end up paying for each procedure. In addition to treating illnesses, doctors must become mini-experts in insurance benefits, out-of-pocket costs, copays, capitation fees, and so on. Medical school and residency teach students to determine the best treatment for patients, but they don't teach students how to make sure that treatment is delivered to the patient, or how to make sure they get paid for their services. Even though most physicians work for practices that have staff for insurance filing, the doctors often must negotiate (and renegotiate) to help their patients get the tests, medications, and so on that they believe are best.

In this way, a physician can't help a patient without understanding the ins and outs of the medical system. Talk about pressure!

For the child who has dreamed of becoming a doctor, the real work begins after completing college. And that's when the stress really starts.

My Dad's Experiences in Medical School and Residency: Thrown into the Fire

Dad didn't have role models for things like how to set boundaries, remain present with family members, or even ask for help. Since he grew up without rules or close family bonds, he instead learned self-reliance. Having no one to ask for help forced my father to find his own way to succeed.

Nowhere was Dad's determination more evident than in his schoolwork. Even though no one nagged him to study or looked over his homework to ensure that he progressed, Dad pushed himself to excel academically.

My father was one of the smartest people I've known. He loved to learn. Even as an adult, he read medical books and journals for fun, not because he had to. And he absolutely loved science. He was an A student because of this, and he was very hard on himself.

Once after getting a B in a class, Dad ran away in seventh grade to Virginia to go be with his biological father Glen. He was not gone long before Grandma Louise retrieved him.

Alongside his academic pursuits, Dad worked as an ambulance driver in high school. His grades earned him admission to Anderson College, a junior college in the upstate now known as Anderson University.

In addition to his love of learning, he loved pranks. He once filled a friend's dorm room with so many balloons that no one could open the door. Another time, he rigged a shaving cream can so when someone opened the door, the can exploded and filled the room. His most infamous prank—and one that got him into the most trouble—was when he and his friends would wrap an unlucky dorm mate into a sheet and toss them from bed to bed. Sadly, once while they were doing this, a dorm mate hit his head on the floor when the pranksters "missed" the bed. The student got a concussion.

As a result of these antics, my grandmother received frequent letters from the school that started with, "We regret to inform you that your son has received demerits for..." or something to that effect. Yes, most of the pranks involved drinking, but my father never got in direct trouble for drinking. Years later I realized that this lifestyle of his was the basis of the advice he gave me when I went off to college. He told me, "Don't let studying get in the way of your college education."

After two years at Anderson College, he transitioned to Clemson University and graduated with a degree in medical technology. He took a job in a pathology lab at a local hospital while applying to medical school at the Medical University of South Carolina. During this time, he met my mom who was working at the same hospital as a phlebotomist. They married six months later in 1969, and he entered medical school soon after. While in medical school, he studied all the time and was the first person ever to earn a perfect score on the pathology exam. My mom said that it was like he was in competition with the professors to be smarter than them. And he loved the challenge. According to my mom, Dad never complained about medical school.

When I went to medical school, my father warned me about the perils of clinical rotations. "Senior residents or attendings will try to humiliate you," he said. "After long hours without sleep, you might be tempted to take something to stay alert. Many of my classmates took speed to remain awake."

"Did you ever do speed?" I asked him.

"No," he smiled. "I relied on good old-fashioned caffeine."

Another time, he gave me the best piece of advice ever, which was that nurses can be "your best friend or worst enemy"—meaning they can help you or hurt you. He explained that "medicine is a team sport, and you must be a team player." I've lived by this rule, and in fact, some of my best friends are nurses.

My dad took a job at Veterans Affairs (VA) doing autopsies during his third year of medical school. Not only did he do it because he needed the money—$50 for each autopsy—but he also loved medicine.

In 1974, he graduated from medical school. I was born that same year.

Next, he interned for a year before heading into private practice. He was what was formerly known as a general practitioner. My father never said much about his internship, but when I later told him about my experiences, he remarked that my internship seemed very different than his. "I rarely saw my supervising attendings (the full-time doctors that supervised the students, interns, and residents)," he told me. "They left me to take care of patients on my own. And we weren't encouraged to call our attendings when we didn't know what to do. If we did, they'd say, 'Figure it out yourself!'" My dad loved that kind of autonomy, and now that I know his history, I understand why.

Students who complete and pass medical school earn their MDs. At that point, they've earned the title of "Doctor." But even after all their years of education, they aren't ready to practice medicine alone. Instead, they enter a hospital system where they are called *interns* (first year of residency) or *residents* (every year after the first year). Interns need more supervision and are often supervised by residents. Interns and residents are both supervised by an attending (a.k.a., a supervising physician) who is ultimately responsible for the decisions made about each patient. They then spend the next three to seven years (depending on their specific program and specialty) working in *residency*. As residents, they work under the license and with close supervision from a board-certified doctor referred to as an *attending* or *supervising physician*.

Why is the term *residents* used in this situation? The practice of formal, on-the-job training for doctors began in the mid-twentieth century. At that time, physicians lived in hospital-supplied housing where they were on call two or three nights a week, for up to three years. Since residents literally lived on-site, they spent all their waking hours in the hospital, treating patients under the "careful supervision" of a skilled doctor (Chiaravalloti 2019).

Residency requirements have changed drastically since my father completed medical school in the 1970s. Back then, residents had no restrictions on the number of hours they would work. Making rounds (the practice of doctors checking in on each of their patients) was brutal. With long hours, huge caseloads, and limited sleep while being fresh out of school, some residents washed out and were therefore seen as "weak."

Instead of using praise or expressing appreciation, many attending physicians relied on statements like, "You should have seen this job back in my day. Things were a helluva lot harder, and we never complained." To this day, you can still hear these statements echoed in the halls of any hospital.

Residents needed to be fully focused and alert despite working forty-eight- or seventy-two-hour days, which led some to substance misuse. Some residents took stimulants to help perk themselves up and alcohol to bring them back down when they had the chance to sleep. The residents that turned to alcohol and drugs did so because of the stigma associated with being viewed as "weak." Given the years that these residents spent completing undergraduate and medical school, they were under immense pressure to avoid "washing out" because they "couldn't keep up" or showed signs of physical or mental distress. Self-medicating became a way to endure the long hours and relentless stress of their job.

No, not every resident of my father's era used stimulants or alcohol to get through grueling times. I don't think my father did during residency (according to my mom), but he did later in life. Eventually, he relied on alcohol to "stabilize" his moods. He kept this drinking hidden from his patients and employers as best as he could. But he also tried to conceal his drinking from his wife (my mother). She came from a conservative Christian background with an alcoholic father, and he didn't want to disappoint her by letting her know of his dependance on alcohol.

A Physician's Sources of Pressure

All jobs have a certain element of stress and pressure, but medical professionals have some unique to their profession.

Sleep Deprivation and Long Hours

Roles where an employee must stay focused and mentally alert as a matter of life and death usually come with safeguards such as these examples from another profession (U.S. Dept. of Transportation 2022). These employees:

- Can work a maximum of eleven hours *only after having ten consecutive hours off.*
- Are required to take a thirty-minute break after eight consecutive hours at work.
- Can work no more than seventy hours each week, *after which they need at least thirty-four hours off before starting the next workweek.*
- Are required to "sleep" (or not work) for ten hours each twenty-four-hour period.

Sadly, these rules don't apply to medical professionals. They apply to truck drivers. A tired truck driver runs the risk of falling asleep behind the wheel, something that could have dire, deadly consequences for others. According to the Federal Motor Carrier Safety Administration, more than 750 people die each year due to fatigued truck drivers. Another 20,000 are injured (Arnold & Itkin 2023).

Let's compare that to residency where, as of 2023, new doctors are limited to eighty hours each week. Eighty hours! Compare that with the thirty-five-hour work week of the average American.

"But at least they get paid well," you might say.

That can be true, but it might not be as much as you think. First year residents earn an average of $55,000 per year (Buga 2021). Let's do the math. Making $55,000 each year while working fifty-two eighty-hour weeks comes to $13.22 per hour. Considering that the average hourly wage in the US is now over $33 per hour, it's inaccurate to say that residents get paid well (YCharts 2023).

When I worked in residency, the eighty-hour work week maximum wasn't enforced. One night, some colleagues and I broke down how many hours we worked each week. We were averaging one hundred hours. Using our salary and the number of hours we averaged, we learned that we as residents made less than minimum wage—which was less than $6 an hour at that time!

After residency and completing the medical boards, residents who choose to work at an academic medical center (AMC) can become *supervising physicians (a.k.a., attendings).* Attending doctors are the senior physicians that oversee the work of a group of residents. Unlike residents, attendings have no limitations on the number of hours they are allowed to work. They work until the job is done and the patients are taken care of.

It's common for attendings to work for thirty-six hours straight without sleep. In fact, some surgeons stay at the hospital for more than three days without going home, and they rely on infrequent catnaps to keep them going. Others, like me, take calls from home after working for eight to twelve hours in the day, at times only getting one to two hours of sleep at a time between addressing phone calls from the hospital, needs of patients, and outside physicians requiring a consult. And I do this for seven days or more at a time!

How comfortable would you feel if you knew the doctor rushing you into surgery hadn't slept for the last thirty-six hours?

Attendings often brag about their lack of sleep and how they spend every other night on call, as those stressors are badges of honor. Calling in sick or asking for help was considered a weakness in the past, and still is by some. Few attendings miss their work shift, mostly because patients don't stop getting sick just because their doctor is sick. Even leaving on time at the end of a long shift can be viewed as a sign of disinterest. The message these behaviors send to residents is this: if you wish to practice medicine, you must be willing to accept the costs.

My father never called in sick unless he was admitted to the hospital. He pressed on when he hadn't slept for days. For him, as it is for many still today, accepting the costs became his way of life, and it changed how he perceived himself and his responsibilities. For example, I visited my parents when I was very pregnant, and I ended up heading to the hospital in premature labor to give birth to his first grandchild. At the same time I left to give birth, Dad headed to work at a different hospital because, as he said to me, "I could not find someone to cover." He continued to work at all costs until the day he died.

Pimping

As if long work hours and life-and-death decision-making weren't brutal enough, historically, residents were often subjected to something called "pimping," the practice of an attending or senior resident asking rapid-fire questions about a patient, disease, or medication until the resident gets an answer wrong or can't answer it. Then, the attending rolls their eyes, belittles the resident, and picks on that resident for the remainder of the day.

Pimping is now less aggressive than it was when my dad attended medical school, but it still existed when I was a resident.

"What is Lasix?" the attending asked me.

"It's a drug used to treat fluid overload. It helps the kidneys make more urine," I answered.

"Where does it work in the body?" the attending asked.

"It works in the thick ascending limb of the loop of Henle in the kidney," I responded, feeling good about correctly answering two questions in a row.

"What transporter does it work on?"

"Sodium-potassium-chloride channel," I answered quickly. I felt good at this point.

"Draw the transporter channel," the attending challenged me.

I didn't know how to do it, which showed on my face.

"No?" the attending asked. "You don't know how to draw it, yet you just prescribed this to a patient?"

Pimping lets an attending show a resident that the attending alone possesses omniscience, whereas the resident, both as an individual and part of a collective, is ignorant. The attendings did this to dominate the students, like a hazing ritual designed to remind the residents that they were at the bottom of the power structure. While some would say they did it to push the resident to study harder, there were ways other than humiliation to accomplish this task.

Most medical school students have been overachievers their entire lives, hearing frequent praise for their accomplishments.

But once a student enters medical school and residency, the praise ends. They are now in an environment where everyone is an overachiever, and excellence is expected.

In some ways, residency is the white-collar equivalent to military boot camp. Both residency and boot camp were designed to dehumanize and humiliate new recruits while instilling them with discipline and the skills they needed to survive. While in boot camp, recruits are called maggots; once recruits complete their training, they earn the title of marine. Similarly, new MDs are called residents. They can't practice medicine except from under the watchful eyes of attendings. They rarely hear praise or encouragement, yet they receive ongoing criticism for every perceived mistake. It's not until residents complete their multi-year residency programs and pass their medical boards that they begin to feel like a "real" doctor.

Since I experienced this kind of behavior from attendings when I served as a resident and fellow, I can only imagine how much worse it would have been for my father before pimping got formally reformed to something gentler. I entered medical school and residency with strong self-esteem, largely due to how my parents had treated me in my childhood. My father didn't have such a supportive upbringing, and he continually fought imposter syndrome and low self-esteem. I have no doubt that the pimping he took from the attendings brought him lower still.

Nowadays the criticism in this scenario is more "sugar-coated." Rather than saying to a resident, "You picked the wrong antibiotic for this patient," they say, "while most of the time the antibiotic that you choose would be correct, in this potential scenario, it does not cover all the possible organisms for this patient. But I'm glad to see that you have learned the most common uses. Good job." This is sandwiching criticism with positives.

Once a resident becomes a real doctor, another physician will leave out any positive words when a peer makes a mistake. Instead, they'll call the "offender" out on it cold. Worse yet, some attendings get so defensive about their mistakes that they'd rather argue than ever admit that they were in the wrong.

Medicine teaches you to be right at all costs. Admitting you're wrong is a sign of weakness—or that you're not as smart as your peers.

Information Overload

The duration of medical school and residency hasn't changed over the decades. However, the amount of information students must learn has grown exponentially. New medicines, diagnostic criteria, technologies, and breakthroughs happen daily, which means new doctors must cram in an ever-expanding amount of knowledge in a fixed amount of time.

After studying pharmacology several years ago, I talked with my dad about some of the medications I'd learned about.

"Now what's that medication do?" my dad asked me.

"It's another hypertensive drug," I told him. "It's one of the dozens on the market."

"When I was in school, I think we had two or three drugs to choose from," my dad smiled.

I had to learn exponentially more about pharmaceuticals than my father learned when he attended medical school. Older doctors must stay current on medical trends and changes, but they don't have to learn it all in one compressed time like new doctors must.

Debt

College isn't cheap. Millions of students enter college and amass large debts along the path to their degrees, because they view college as an investment. The estimated annual cost of college projected for 2025 is as follows (MEFA 2023):

National Public 4-Year In-State Tuition	National Public 4-Year Out-of-State Tuition	National Private 4-Year
$25,406.43	$44,310.61	$58,384.51

In pursuit of obtaining a bachelor's degree, the average student borrows more than $30,000. And even twenty years after entering college, half of all students still owe an average of $20,000 in loan debt (Hanson 2023).

While that's a lot of debt, the figures are significantly higher for medical school graduates. In 2023, the average cost of medical school reached $300,000 (Asch et. Al 2020). On average, students amass more than $250,000 in student loan debt while in medical school, and more than 40 percent of those students also carry premedical educational debts. The average medical student owes seven times more than a typical college graduate.

For medical students and residents, time is not on their side. Most will reach age thirty-six before they complete their residency programs, pass their medical boards, and receive compensation as fully licensed doctors. Meanwhile, those who completed college with undergraduate degrees at twenty-two have had fourteen years to start paying off student loans, buying homes, saving, and investing in their retirement accounts. While serving as residents, their medical school student debt interest is deferred, but undergraduate school loans keep accumulating interest (Medical Economics 2019).

If you were to invest $20,000 at age twenty-two for forty years with an average annual return of 6 percent, that investment would grow to more than $205,000 by the time you reached sixty-two.

Let's compare that same $20,000 investment at age thirty-six, the age when most residents become fully licensed doctors. Since doctors start saving later, they have only twenty-six years before reaching age sixty-two. Using the same average annual return of 6 percent, their $20,000 investment would grow to less than $91,000.

While physicians ultimately make good money, the time to let their money work for them is not on their side.

Death, Depression, Addiction, and Suicide

At this point, you may be thinking, *With all of these negative factors, why should I pursue a career in medicine?* I understand the sentiment, but I'd like to clarify that my goal isn't to steer you away from becoming a physician. There are many pluses, as you know—which (I assume) is why you're entering the field or considering doing so. Rather than dissuade you, I want to equip you on how to navigate the stresses that you may not hear about as you prepare for medical school. And I want to provide you with some tools to make your experience more positive and healthier than the doctors of yesteryear—including my father.

On that note, in Chapter 1, I shared how adults who suffered adverse childhood experiences (ACEs) are more susceptible to future physical and mental health problems. The stress of residency can be especially crippling for young doctors who lived through ACEs. However, stress doesn't only affect doctors at risk from childhood traumas. It also affects doctors who must endure: long work hours that require continuous focus. Sleep deprivation. Pimping from attendings. Growing debt.

But let's not forget the stress that comes with the job.

Death. Residents see dozens of patients each day, people with different conditions, medications, and prognoses. Throughout medical school, the concepts of life and death remained mostly in the abstract. Doctors-in-training read books and sat through lectures about various diseases that could take a person's life. In residency, though, death becomes real, inescapable, and personal. Residents build bonds with patients who laugh, dream, love, and experience life. And then some of those patients die.

A first-year resident had this to say about the most difficult part of the job: "I had a patient who coded pretty early on in my intern year. I had been taking care of him for a week, and it was difficult because I had grown close to him. I didn't handle it very well because I blamed myself." (Brown 2021).

Medical school trains doctors to diagnose and treat patients' health problems; however, medical school doesn't really prepare doctors to confront death on a regular basis. The COVID-19 pandemic only exaggerated this gap in their experience. Doctors were not prepared to see multiple patients dying every single day.

Depression. In one study, nearly 10 percent of first year residents reported feeling depressive symptoms.

But the actual number is darker still. When researchers conducted an anonymous, confidential survey of residents, nearly one-half of first-year residents self-reported symptoms compatible with severe depression. Additionally, nearly 25 percent reported having suicidal ideation (Mian et al. 2018).

Students attracted to medicine often expect themselves to be perfect. With that in mind, it's not surprising that only 1 percent of residents decide to take a leave for "emotional reasons." Of those who take leave, some are admitted into psychiatric facilities, attempt suicide, or receive treatment for addiction (Goebert et al. 2009).

Stress takes a greater toll on female residents than males. Due to traditional gender roles, female residents are more likely to report challenges with stress related to the competing demands of home, family, and work. Additionally, females often find that their higher education and career goals limit their ability to attract and date non-physician partners. Many males still find the idea of woman making more money than they do as a threat to the traditional concept that men (not women) should be the main breadwinner in the household. Finally, a large number of female doctors express concerns about delaying the start of their own families (Sanfey et al. 2015).

Untreated depressive episodes can lead to impaired decision-making. A cross-sectional study of medical students estimates up to 18 percent of students show signs of impaired professional decision-making and skills. When those with signs of impaired judgment were asked if they would voluntarily seek help, the majority declined, citing fear (Primack et al. 2010) (more on this later).

Addiction. Addiction goes underreported within the medical community. Estimates suggest that doctors are thirty to one hundred times more likely to suffer from an addiction than the general population. Another study showed that "heavy drug use, including use of alcohol," was 1.6 times greater than in the general population.

A resident-specific survey revealed the "drugs of choice" for residents: Eleven percent used tranquilizers and 9 percent used opiates. In a separate confidential survey, residents reported that once they received prescribing privileges, many wrote their own prescriptions for benzodiazepines and prescription opiates. While physicians can no longer self-prescribe controlled medications in the US, the internet has made it so they don't need to. The black market offers an array of controlled medications that can be shipped right to your house. Sadder still, nearly 10 percent of doctors with addiction attempt, or die, by suicide.

Suicide. Undiagnosed and untreated depression can be fatal. The suicide rate for medical students is nearly three times higher than for others in the same-age college cohort. Suicide is the second leading cause of death for medical students (accidents are number one). The number of suicides is likely underreported. Some of the "accidents" are suicides that are covered up or mislabeled. Data on the leading causes of residents' deaths tells a similar story. Death by suicide is the second highest cause of death for residents (trailed only by malignant neoplasm).

Remember that some doctors already have some of these challenges before they start medical school. Yet there are other students who enter the medical field with no propensity for depression, addiction, or suicidal thoughts, and these students can still develop problems once they join the healthcare field. Those who develop troubles as students and residents won't easily reset their behavior patterns once they serve as licensed doctors, unless they seek intervention.

Surviving the Stress of Medical School and Residency

This all implies that even doctors who came from happy, supportive homes and show no signs of depression, addiction, or suicidal ideation aren't immune from struggles. At some point in medical school, all students feel the weight of information overload. All but the wealthiest medical school graduates (and those with no financial concerns are the vast minority) will incur student debt. Then in residency, all doctors experience the stress of working relentless, long hours with intense focus. All will endure some level of pimping, even though this once-common practice has diminished somewhat. And some will face an existential crisis when they first confront the death of a patient. Many residents experience depression, and some fall into addictions. Some even decide to end their lives before they practice medicine under their own licenses.

But students and residents can develop healthy habits to get them through these most challenging learning periods. Following are some habits that I recommend. Many of these strategies apply even after residency but developing them early on will help you as you transition into the rest of your career.

Enter Counselling

The Center for Disease Control (CDC) reports that nearly 10 percent of adults in the US sought mental health treatment in 2019 (Terlizzi and Zablotsky 2020). In my opinion, that number should be higher. In fact, I believe that everyone can benefit from talking regularly with a neutral, trained therapist. Creating this habit early —even before entering medical school or at the first sign of high stress—can help someone develop skills for the long-haul. Think of it like going to the doctor when you notice a suspicious spot on your skin; you want to get it examined, biopsied, and treated before any potential malignancy takes over.

Therapy offers more than validation for a person's feelings. A skilled therapist can also provide you a safe place to vent negative emotions, acquire new life skills, learn tips for emotional regulation, assist in self-discovery, and help eliminate self-defeating thoughts and behaviors. Most therapists can also help you assess how any ACEs you experienced might be driving your emotions and behaviors, which can lead to breakthroughs in relationships and resiliency.

A former therapist friend of mine told me that each time he experienced the death of a client, his organization mandated that he see a counsellor before returning to work. Police officers who fire a gun in the line of duty must do the same. These mandatory safeguards exist to ensure the well-being of the counselor and police officers. While physicians don't currently have this requirement, I believe they should.

Practice Mindfulness

One resident described what residency feels like by saying this: "As resident physicians, some of us tend to make it seem like we're floating along peacefully. But, early on we're all like ducks; we may look fine on the surface, but we're paddling like crazy below the water."

Mindfulness is the basic human ability to be fully present, aware of where we are and what we're doing, and not overly reactive or overwhelmed by what's going on around us (Mindfulness.com 2022).

Mindfulness helps you recharge after being constantly alert for long, stressful hours. Mindfulness can slow down your world, so you no longer feel like you're "paddling like crazy."

Almost any activity can help you tap into the benefits of mindfulness as long as you're focusing on what you're doing, and you're bringing all your senses into play. Take gardening as an example of a simple activity that can bring you into a state of mindfulness. You see, touch, and smell the soil. While working in the garden, you can hear insects and birds. Even if you have only five minutes away to pull weeds in a small patch of your garden, you gain a sense of accomplishment for what you've completed.

Meditation is a mindfulness activity with many health benefits, according to numerous studies. Focusing on your breath and slowing it down takes practice, but doing so can help you take a mental "time out" in any stressful situation—breathing to re-regulate your parasympathetic nervous system. When you operate from a calm state, not only can you make better decisions, but you likely will also be paying your body a favor by reducing its cortisol and other stress hormones.

As we know, long-term, heightened stress can wreak havoc on health, so managing your stress response is a highly valuable skill. There are numerous meditation and mindfulness apps and tools available to help you get started on building your stress-reducing muscles.

View Residency as an Extension of Medical School

Apprenticeships involve both classroom learning and on-the-job training. It generally takes around four to five years to become a licensed plumber or a licensed electrician. During those years, apprentices experience the real-world work of those professions.

Similar to an apprenticeship, a residency is the on-the-job training portion of your education. If you start your internship believing that you've already learned everything in medical school, you'll be in for a huge shock.

One resident shared this about his residency experience: "The more you learn in residency, the more you realize how much you don't know." Another shared a similar view: "It's OK to not know everything....You're not really expected to know everything and be perfectly right from the get-go. It's a huge learning process. There's a steep learning curve, and you'll eventually get there."

If you enter residency believing you must know everything, you'll add unnecessary stress to an already stressful job. If you view residency as an extension of medical school, you'll have an easier time pacing yourself for the long haul.

Mandated Debriefs After a Patient's Death

While this strategy isn't something you control as a resident, I'm including it here because I think it's important for physicians and leaders to consider—especially as it pertains to residents.

Doctors must walk a fine line between empathizing with patients and their families and remaining emotionally detached. This is an art, not one that all doctors master. If a doctor cares too personally and deeply for the suffering of a patient, the doctor will fall apart after every loss. If a doctor doesn't empathize with what each patient and their family are enduring, that physician will come across as being cold and uncaring.

I believe one way to help new doctors find the balance is to hold a debrief after the death of a patient. I'm not suggesting a clinical debrief where the team tries to determine what, if anything, could have saved the patient. Rather I'm referring to debriefing the emotions a resident and the care team feel after each loss. Give them space to share their feelings.

A healthcare consultant friend of mine told me about attending his first "Reading of the Names" meeting he attended. This was a monthly meeting held at a hospice group he supported. The names were of the patients who died during the previous month.

He said that the nurse began the meeting by telling the all-employee group that 127 people had died under their organization's care over the past month. My friend said, "At first, I cringed inside, thinking, *They're going to read 127 names? This is going to take forever!* But as the nurse slowly read each name, I settled down and began to process what I was hearing. In no time, I switched off the business consultant part of my brain, and my human side—the side with my own elderly father and mother—took over." As the nurse continued reading, he said he thought of each name as a person with hopes, dreams, favorite foods, friendships, family members, and full lives that were not over. He began to cry. He had never met a single patient, yet he pictured what their lives must have been like, and he started to mourn for those he had never met.

"What surprised me the most," he continued, "was that several of the hundreds of staff members in the room either had tears in their eyes or rolling down their faces. The executive director sat in the back of the room, and I could see him wiping his eyes. They didn't try to detach from their emotions. Instead, they embraced them. And after a patient died, they changed out the bed linen while weeping. Then they oversaw the next dying patient checking into the room. And they did this repeatedly, with no less compassion each time."

My friend concluded that these hospice workers offered their patients two things: pain management and love. Since curing the dying wasn't an option, these workers allowed themselves to love and feel fully instead of treating their patients like numbers. And the compassion they showed was reflected in the organization's unmatched reputation in the community. Healthcare leaders take note: this kind of patient-centric approach can pay off in terms of referrals, reputation, and decreased time spent managing complaints or disputes.

I'm not suggesting that your department or team of physicians must weep over every loss. But if we follow the example of this hospice organization, we can learn that recognizing a death can be a positive experience for a culture and the individuals within it. It reinforces both the patient and caregiver as individual human beings with whole lives and emotions.

While many residency programs encourage or require these debriefs, I believe they should be mandatory for all. Even the programs that mandate such sessions don't require the attending physician to be present. This is a mistake. Who better than the attending to show residents that it's acceptable to grieve the loss of a patient? When an attending takes part in a debrief after a death, their presence shows the resident the very human side of patient care. The physician can also model a healthy and appropriate way to show this grief, so that it doesn't negatively impact day-to-day operations.

Work With a Financial Planner

When I was in medical school, several financial planners offered free sessions to students. As I recall, few students took advantage of those offers. That's a shame, since every medical school student I've known carries debt from student loans. The sooner they get guidance, the sooner they'll climb out of debt and start investing for their futures.

As Steve Booren, author of *Blind Spots: The Mental Mistakes Investors Make*, states about investing, "Start early and save consistently throughout your career....If you want the ability to make choices about what you do with your time, your interests, and your relationships, start now. The real reason for saving and accumulating wealth is freedom. And freedom, like prosperity, is a mindset." As most investment experts will tell you, the time spent "in the market" is the best indicator of how much those investments will earn over your lifetime. When you're also managing debt at the start of your career, this is a balancing act you'll want to discover.

A *financial planner* is someone who can advise you on topics like budgeting, savings strategies, and managing debt. You may also want a *financial advisor* who can help you with a broader range of financial needs, including insurance recommendations and overseeing your investments. Many financial advisors are also certified financial planners (CFPs) or chartered financial analysts (CFAs). Some financial advisors charge a percentage of your portfolio each year, while others charge a flat fee, so explore their pricing options—and thoroughly vet any professional you're thinking of using. Consider also reading books about investments to learn more.

Ask the doctors around you for recommendations to find the best financial planner or financial advisor. Some work exclusively with doctors. Interview various professionals to find one who will help you realize your financial goals.

Starting to work with a planner or an advisor while you're in medical school or your residency will ensure that you're prepared as you transition from carrying debt with no or little income, to earning a regular salary. Doing so will eliminate some of the stress you feel when you see the interest on your undergraduate student loan debts increasing.

Protect Your Downtime

Some people, like my father, have an abundance of energy. These folks feel the need to keep busy and move all the time. Even those of us with less vigor can turn into the "Energizer bunny" when we're excited about what we're doing and having fun. Perhaps that's why some first-year residents find the pace of residency exhilarating and energizing...at first. But there's a reason why so many first-year residents experience depression.

Your residency schedule will change regularly, but that doesn't mean you can't make plans; rather, it requires that you make plans that are flexible so you can safeguard your time off. Remind yourself that your residency is a marathon, not a sprint. If you start at a pace that is too fast, you may not have the endurance for the three to seven years that lie ahead.

One resident had this to say about the importance of stepping away from work: "Take your day off to wind down and do something you enjoy. Doing this helps you come back to work for the following week refreshed, and you don't have the lingering exhaustion and unresolved feelings from the prior week."

Another shared about how important they found it to get proper rest: "Sleep is one of the best medicines. Make it a priority to get seven hours a night." (Note that most sleep experts recommend eight, not seven, hours of uninterrupted sleep each night).

Along those same thoughts, another resident suggested this: "Find a few minutes for yourself or your family to step away from medicine, allow your mind to recharge, and then come back into it."

Still another suggested, "Make sure to get regular exercise. It sounds simple, and we know this since we're trained medical professionals, but it's easy to let our physical health slide when we're exhausted. I go to the gym in the morning, and I try to fit in a game of tennis with friends on the weekend. On days I can't do any formal exercise, I at least take a walk after dinner." Besides making you physically stronger and healthier, as you know, exercise releases endorphins which can help you combat stress.

Those who grew up with a nine-to-five Monday through Friday mindset might find it challenging to not have evenings and every weekend off. Instead of waiting for a long, solid block of time to decompress, the residents that do the best know how to take advantage of every minute of downtime afforded them.

Stay Socially Connected

Extroverts recharge their batteries by being around other people. Introverts, on the other hand, get the same energy from downtime spent alone or with another introverted person; but research has shown repeatedly that both introverts and extroverts benefit from staying socially connected.

Even though I've spent years prescribing various medications for health issues, I understand that not every condition requires a prescription. People with strong social connections experience lower rates of anxiety and depression, higher self-esteem, greater empathy, and stronger relationships—all of which can strengthen their immune systems, help them recover from sickness, and may even promote longevity (Victoria Dept. of Health & Human Services 2017).

I can't think of any medication with so many positive benefits and no negative side effects.

Long hours and irregular schedules make it difficult to maintain and build strong connections with others. Many residents become friends with other residents, since both parties understand the stress of the job. I developed several close relationships with my fellow residents, and some of them remain in my support network years later.

But not all relationships are beneficial to your well-being. Home organization expert Marie Kondo has written several books about tidying up your home. When helping people decide if they should keep or discard an item during the tidying up process, she suggests that people hold an item and ask themselves, "Does this spark joy?" If it doesn't spark joy, she encourages people to get rid of the item (Malito 2019). Practice the same concept with the people you choose to spend time with. No, you can't discard patients or bosses that don't "spark joy" in you. But you can choose the people you spend time with when you're not working. If you spend time with negative, critical people, they will rub off on you. Similarly, when you spend time with those who are supportive, loving, kind, and compassionate, those traits will also transfer to you.

Develop and Use a Mantra

A mantra is a short, simple, "sticky" saying that a person can repeat when times get difficult. One of my favorite mantras comes from a Persian proverb: *This too shall pass.*

What I love about this mantra is its two-fold meaning. The first is obvious. When you face a challenge, remind yourself that no problem lasts forever. The second meaning is less overt. *This too shall pass* is a way to remind yourself to stay mindful of the best moments in your life, because good times, just like bad ones, won't last forever. When you feel crushed by the weight of stress, lean into the happy times you've experienced.

Whatever mantra you use, repeat it often enough to yourself that you believe it and take strength from it.

Chapter 2 Summary

Medical school and residency are challenging. You must remain mentally sharp and focused at all times. Additionally, you must work long hours while sleep deprived. While the conditions have improved, you'll still experience some form of pimping from your attendings. And let's not forget about the constant nagging in the back of your mind about the amount debt you're carrying.

Many residents experience stress from the job itself. Doctors aren't trained in how to handle the death of patients. Many residents struggle from situational depression, and some even turn to an addiction to alcohol or drugs as they attempt to self-medicate away bad feelings and shut down their minds so they can sleep. And sadly, some feel suicidal and act upon those feelings.

While it's not easy, you can survive this prolonged trial by fire through implementing these best practices:

- Enter counselling
- Practice mindfulness

- View residency as an extension of medical school
- Work with a financial planner to relieve any pressure you feel about debt
- Protect your downtime
- Stay socially connected
- Develop and use a mantra to repeat during trying times

In the next chapter, I will share some of the challenges doctors face once they leave residency.

Receiving Your Medical License: Out of the Frying Pan and into the Fire

I haven't shared all the hoops that would-be doctors must jump through to become licensed physicians. If you're already a doctor, you have experienced these steps firsthand. If you're a resident, as we discussed in the last chapter, some of these are already behind you. But if you're in the exploratory phase of considering a career as a medical doctor, let me back up and give you the high-level overview of the steps involved before you can practice medicine.

First, complete undergraduate school. You'll likely pursue a degree in pre-med, biology (or biological sciences), exercise science, or similar course work that meets the prerequisite science courses and labs required by many medical schools. During your junior year, you'll need to register for and take the Medical College Admission Test (MCAT), which is the standardized examination used by medical school admission committees to assess the likelihood that you'll do well in medical school. A good MCAT score is 511 or higher, with the highest possible score of 528. Of the two hundred thousand students taking the MCAT each year, only thirty to seventy students achieve a perfect score (Kaplan 2023).

If you get a good score on the MCAT, it's time to apply to medical schools—while you're still completing your undergraduate degree. The average medical school applicant applies to sixteen different schools (Shemmassian 2023). Applying to too few schools means you might not find a good fit. Conversely, applying to too many schools is very expensive, since in addition to application fees, students must pay out-of-pocket when traveling to interviews.

Once you're accepted into medical school, plan on being a full-time student for another four years. Your time will be divided between classroom instruction and clinical rotations for field experience. While in medical school, you'll need to take and receive a passing score on each part of the United States Medical Licensing Examination (USMLE), a three-part examination. Students are required to pass the first part of the examination prior to entering their third year of medical school, the second part of the exam during their fourth year of medical school, and the third part prior to finishing residency.

Not surprisingly, the competition to get into medical school is huge. Schools examine several variables when considering who they will accept into their programs, since it's in the best interest of the institution and the student to select those with the greatest chance of successfully completing their programs.

Still, between 15.7 and 18.4 percent of students drop out of medical school without completing their degrees. Interestingly though, those who drop out typically do so for non-academic reasons, such as entering medical school with overconfidence, failing to build relationships with fellow students and faculty, experiencing family stressors, or deciding that medicine isn't the right career choice (Ponio 2023).

Towards the end of medical school, you'll need to find a residency program in your medical specialty of interest. If you're fortunate enough to find a residency match, you'll spend the next three to eight years in residency. For example: Surgical residencies are a minimum of five years. Oral and maxillofacial surgery residents need to complete a four-year graduate degree in dentistry plus a minimum of four years in a general surgery training program. (ACS 2023).

How hard is it to find a residency program? Currently, due to capacity issues, only 75 percent of qualified medical school graduates have a residency position they can land in.

So...no pressure, right? Even with a medical degree and eight years of college, around 8,600 doctors don't find a residency match on their first attempt (Finnegan 2016).

Even if you land a coveted residency program, it's not time to rest quite yet! After completing these steps, you still must get ready for board certification. This written exam may include an oral portion as well. The test evaluates doctor readiness in six competencies:

1. Practice-based learning and improvement

2. Patient care and procedural skills
3. Systems-based practice
4. Medical knowledge
5. Interpersonal and communication skills
6. Professionalism

After this exam, you're almost there. The last step is to get a state license to practice medicine and a federal license to dispense medications. Each state sets its own licensing requirements and procedures, so you'll need to investigate how to obtain licensure in whatever state you intend to set up shop.

Whew! You've been a diligent student throughout high school, college, medical school, residency, the USMLE, and board certification. You likely missed out on some of the fun that others experienced during their time in school. You've probably amassed more than a quarter of a million dollars in debt. By this point, you're exhilarated to be done with school. Your sacrifice, long hours, and resilience have gotten you this far.

By now, you're probably in your early to mid-thirties. Yet you still don't have a job or earn a paycheck.

Congratulations! You've just moved from the frying pan into the fire.

My Father Had No Road Map for Doctoring

After Dad completed his schooling and other requirements, he decided to settle in Lake View, South Carolina. He arrived in Lake View during the seventies when the population had reached its apex at just under a thousand people. He chose Lake View when the town leaders agreed to build him an office and pay some of his debt in a sort of indentured servitude arrangement that worked for both parties.

When he opened his medical practice, he was the only primary care physician in the town. Already married with two children, Dad took this route to provide some stability to his family. But having a "monopoly" came at a price. Dad worked all the time. He would leave to make rounds at the hospital before I awoke. Then he would head to his office where he saw patients all day. Before going home, he would return to do rounds once again at the hospital.

"Hey Dr. T," people shouted and waved whenever I walked in town with Dad. "You got a minute?" He couldn't step outside without someone coming over to chat with him. People weren't stopping him for free medical advice on the sidewalk. Most of them just wanted to talk with him, shake his hand, and express their appreciation that he had come to Lake View. And of course, I loved being the daughter of a celebrity. Little did I know that Dad was unhappy. My mother was unhappy too. And I didn't know until years later how much financial strain my father's early years in medicine put on him.

As his career progressed, Dad's workdays started earlier and continued later, and he spent even less time at home. He would ask Mom to keep us awake so he could spend some time with us when he got home, but we were usually long asleep before he returned.

Many local residents didn't see a doctor unless they were seriously ill. They were put off by the "long drive" (about ten miles away) to the next town to see one, so my dad's clinic was where they all went. Once word got around how "wonderful Dr. T is, You must make an appointment!" people started making more regular appointments. My dad's days became so brutally long that he recruited other physicians to the practice—hoping he could get some downtime. But that failed, because my father was *too good* of a doctor. The people in town all wanted to see "Dr. T." Eventually, he resigned himself to serving out his time-based contract by himself.

Once he completed his time in Lake View, Dad moved us to Dillon, South Carolina, a small town about ten minutes away. Dillon was a slightly bigger version of Lake View, with several doctors' offices and a hospital. My dad opted to try something new, so he exited private practice and started working in the emergency room at the hospital. The "ER" was simply a room with a few bays surrounded by curtains. They had no actual emergency department (ED). It wasn't until 1979 that emergency medicine was approved as a specialty by the American Board of Medical Specialties. The American Board of Emergency Medicine was the independent certifying body for this specialty, and the first certification exam was given in 1980. It wasn't until many years later that most EDs started requiring physicians to be board certified in Emergency Medicine. So of course, Dad hadn't received special training or a board certification for a program that just started (my father started in the ED in the early 80s. Later though, the certification committee offered to "grandfather" Dad into obtaining his board certification, but he never saw the point in getting it. He felt that board certification was just another way for the medical community to get money from him. Some cautioned him that he would regret not getting it, but he never did.)

Like many new doctors, my father had no experience running a small business, which added to his challenges. Medical school prepared him to manage patients for issues like hypertension and pneumonia, but he received no education on money management or business 101. He had to figure out how to order supplies for his "department" and make sure he had the necessary tools to do his job.

Looking back at my own path to practicing medicine, I took physics and organic chemistry, but I was never required to take a business or accounting class. I graduated with a much higher than average earning potential, yet I had no idea of how to deal with money. While many physicians today operate in a larger hospital or healthcare system that manages the organization's finances and administration, most doctors would benefit from at least a cursory knowledge of how these areas work. When requesting supplies or advocating for a new piece of equipment, most chief financial officers (CFOs) appreciate a physician who can make a solid and financially-backed business case for the addition.

As I have shared, adults react to present-day trauma, stress, and adversity the same way they dealt with those challenges in childhood —until they learn otherwise and consciously make new choices. Those exposed to adverse childhood events (ACEs) who don't learn healthy coping mechanisms will continue to struggle as adults. When my father came under pressure, he too reverted to the pattern he developed in childhood, which included isolation and alcohol.

After Residency, Doctors Fly Solo

As tough as medical school and residency can be on doctors, another stressor kicks in when doctors transition from residency to serving as full-time physicians.

No More Safety Net

Throughout residency, doctors have training wheels. Even with their heads full of knowledge, they remain under the watchful eyes of attendings who ensure patient safety. While in residency, doctors have an extra brain, set of eyes, and pair of hands to guide them.

But that umbrella of protection disappears after residency. While few doctors miss the oversight (and sometimes micromanagement) of attendings, once a doctor is on their own, they experience an entirely deeper and more profound sense of responsibility for their patients. Even if they work under a department head, they still retain much more autonomy than they did as residents.

Finding a Job

All the years of preparation mean nothing unless the newly minted doctor finds a place to practice medicine.

If you think back to a time when you've been in job search mode, you remember the stress, insecurity, and fear. Finding a job is like a courtship. You're not only looking for something that makes you happy, but you're looking for a good fit for both you and your potential partner. A job search puts you in perpetual dating mode where you must always bring your best self forward or risk rejection.

Many doctors start their searches during residency. Many stay on at the same facility, transitioning from resident to a full-time position. Others choose to hit the open market for their job searches. And some work with a recruiter to secure positions. But no matter which job search path they take, they can expect to experience some tension.

Taking 100 Percent Responsibility for Patient Outcomes

After residency, new doctors often feel the full weight of responsibility for the health and well-being of their patients.

Even people outside of medicine have heard of the Hippocratic Oath that some institutions still ask doctors to take when they start practicing medicine. "First, do no harm," wasn't included in what we call the Hippocratic Oath. While Hippocrates, considered "the father of Western medicine," wrote these words, they don't actually appear in his Hippocratic Oath.

Instead of taking the Hippocratic Oath, many institutions follow the newly revised version of the Declaration of Geneva adopted in 1948 by the World Medical Association General Assembly and most recently revised on October 14, 2017. Here's what that declaration says:

As a member of the medical profession:

I solemnly pledge to dedicate my life to the service of humanity;

The health and well-being of my patient will be my first consideration;

I will respect the autonomy and dignity of my patient;

I will maintain the utmost respect for human life;

I will not permit considerations of age, disease or disability, creed, ethnic origin, gender, nationality, political affiliation, race, sexual orientation, social standing, or any other factor to intervene between my duty and my patient;

I will respect the secrets that are confided in me, even after the patient has died;

I will practice my profession with conscience and dignity and in accordance with good medical practice;

I will foster the honor and noble traditions of the medical profession;

I will give to my teachers, colleagues, and students the respect and gratitude that is their due;

I will share my medical knowledge for the benefit of the patient and the advancement of healthcare;

I will attend to my own health, well-being, and abilities in order to provide care of the highest standard;

I will not use my medical knowledge to violate human rights and civil liberties, even under threat;

I make these promises solemnly, freely, and upon my honor.

Think about the responsibility resting on a doctor who commits to this line: *As a member of the medical profession, the health and well-being of my patient will be my first consideration.* This oath, when taken literally, means that *being a doctor comes before all else, even before our own physical and mental health.* This oath suggests that as a doctor, you *and you alone* are accountable for all patient outcomes. This is a heavy burden for anyone to carry.

Following are a few additional challenges that doctors face once they become full-fledged, practicing, licensed doctors.

Administrative Duties

While many organizations tout "patients before paperwork," doctors face mountains of administrative responsibilities that have little to do with patient care. Instead of treating clients, physicians spend an inordinate amount of time entering notes into electronic health records, managing insurance issues, delivering test results, and other non-clinical duties.

Practice Management

In addition to administrative duties, many physicians get bogged down with work of managing the practice. Instead of seeing patients, doctors spend time ordering supplies, maintaining and administering information technology, communicating with staff, and managing the overall business.

Patient Outcomes Despite Obstacles

The government imposes quality standards for care that are linked to state and federal reimbursement money for Medicaid and Medicare. Quality is a great thing. Unfortunately, however, some of these "quality" metrics don't take factors outside of the doctor's control into consideration.

Take patients on dialysis for kidney failure, for example. We as doctors must monitor and report hemoglobin and phosphorus levels. But as a physician, I have no control over patients who cancel multiple appointments, causing their hemoglobin levels to drop. Nor do I have control over a patient who continues to eat foods high in phosphorus.

The government also sets a goal for a certain percentage of patients being on home dialysis. Those numbers are difficult to reach when you work in a low socio-economic dialysis unit. For example, patients who haven't finished high school or live in an apartment with ten other people aren't good candidates for home dialysis. Yet the standards leave no room for such outside factors. This puts the responsibility for quality solely on the physicians, or the health-care system, and the patients are not responsible for taking any of that responsibility. To try to meet these standards, physicians must spend extra time with those patients to get them to do what they're supposed to do—or figure out why they're not doing what they're supposed to do. This time is not reimbursed.

Can you imagine an attorney counseling a patient for free?

Patient Advocacy

Doctors spend countless hours learning about the best medications to treat various illnesses and diseases. A doctor wishing to put the *health and well-being* of a patient first may prescribe a specific medication to treat the problem.

And then the insurance company of the patient says no.

A friend of mine recently changed health insurance carriers, moving from the oldest, most patient-centric company to another national carrier. When his doctor prescribed gabapentin for arthritis in his spine, the insurance company refused to cover it. The doctor's office spent a month going back and forth with the insurance company to "prove" that this medication was needed.

Due to undesired side effects, my friend couldn't tolerate gabapentin, so his doctor gave him a prescription for pregabalin. Can you guess what his insurance company said? "No," once again.

The last time I spoke with him, the discussions between his doctor's office and his insurance company have yet to resolve the issue and cover his medication. In the meantime, my friend is in constant pain.

Patients aren't the only ones inconvenienced when insurance companies second-guess doctors. Providers get put in the middle of advocating for their patients with the insurance companies after hours.

This back-and-forth between insurance carriers and providers has been around ever since the health insurance companies created the concept of health plan formularies. Much of the time, doctors must document why one medication should be used over another on a case-by-case basis. Some insurance policies require that a patient try multiple medications before they will approve the one that the doctor believes will actually help. Meanwhile, a patient may be suffering because they don't have the medication they need, and the doctor who's advocating for the patient must jump through additional, time-consuming hoops to solve the problem. This process, and the communication involved with it, takes time.

Suggestions for New Doctors

The transition from resident to full-time doctor can feel like a huge change. For this reason, I usually make time to share with new doctors some of the lessons I learned when I began practicing under my own medical license. Here's my quick list of hacks to make the process smoother and more fulfilling:

- **Wear comfortable shoes.** Just like in residency, you'll be on your feet for hours each day.
- **Find your own physician.** Too many physicians try to serve as their own doctor. Don't make that mistake. Find someone

you trust to serve as your doctor and let that person care for you.

- **Use mentors.** The best way to make it through medical school and residency is to find a mentor. Don't be surprised if you don't find one mentor to guide you in every area you wish to master. For example, you might find a mentor with an enviable bedside manner, another with keen medical insight, and yet another who demonstrates outstanding work-life balance. Instead of simply copying someone who offers some of the traits you want to acquire, look for individuals who get you closer to practicing medicine the way you envision.

- **Develop strong work relationships.** Knowledge is but one piece of what makes you successful as a physician. The best doctors have strong interpersonal skills and are adept at building relationships. Physicians need a solid front- and back-office staff, lab technicians, nurses, social workers, and others to care for patients. In larger practices or hospital systems, they may need to communicate with department heads or chiefs (from their or another department), other c-suite leaders—like a chief medical officer (CMO) or chief executive officer (CEO)—and even a board of directors. From time to time, they may need to ask for favors from staff members within various areas, or advocate for an important change from a higher-level leader. In these ways, your interpersonal and relationship-building skills can make the difference between fair and outstanding patient outcomes—while also improving your workplace culture.

Imagine you're seeing a patient with newly diagnosed hypertension. You did a kidney ultrasound as part of the work-up and also noticed that the patient has multiple cysts on both kidneys. You ask the patient to go to the lab to have blood drawn, but it's now 5 p.m. and the lab is closed. Your nurse agrees to draw the blood for you, and a front desk staff member offers to run it to the local hospital to be processed on their way home.

Doctors need a strong team. Otherwise, patients will be put in the middle and left to navigate the system alone.

- **Use your whole village.** Just like you need fellow professionals to maximize your medical outcomes, you need people outside of work to ground you. Find the balance between *living to work* and *working to live.* Your overall quality of life has less to do with where you practice medicine than with those you spend time with when the workday is complete.

Besides these simple suggestions, Following are some additional ideas to help you transition from residency to serving as a licensed physician.

Protect Yourself

Once you become an attending, you'll be offered many opportunities to get involved with committees, teaching, project development, advocacy, and so on. But these opportunities are not *instead of* but *in addition to* your clinical duties. While some of these opportunities are worth considering, in the beginning, don't take on more than you can handle. You don't want to spend your precious off hours doing extra work. Instead, take a nap or a walk, spend time with your loved ones, or recharge your battery.

Protect Your Off Time (In Other Words, Value Your Work-Life Balance)

As discussed in Chapter 2 about navigating residency, once you're a licensed physician, you must continue to take care of yourself. If you're a parent and/or a spouse, make sure you take time to look after *you*. You have probably heard the saying, "I need a vacation from my vacation." If you're stressed after time off, then is it really time off? Are you trading one stress for another? Make sure your away time is really *away*. I have learned a lot about this from others. I had an attending in fellowship who got a massage after every service week. I have a colleague who takes time for herself twice a year by going away for a weekend and leaving the kids with her husband. She goes to a hotel (even if just locally), eats dinner, and goes to a movie alone. By taking the downtime she needs, she can stay sharp at work and attentive at home.

Practice Time Management

As an attending, you'll be pulled in multiple directions all the time, especially as you assume more administrative and/or teaching duties. If you're all over the place, tasks will take longer to complete. Following are some time management hacks that have helped me:

- Start your day with a plan, writing down everything you need to accomplish, and check items off as you complete each task. Checking off each task once completed gives you a sense of accomplishment and motivates you to complete the next.
- Next, go through your email, and handle all immediate concerns.
- Take a few minutes for lunch each day doing something other than work. I usually surf the web, look at yahoo news, or look at the latest cryptocurrency values. Even if it is only 10 minutes, it helps to reset my brain.
- Each Friday, spend thirty minutes updating your CV with any highlights from your week, if applicable. This will prevent

you from being overwhelmed when someone asks to see it, or you apply for a new role and find it outdated.

Hold Realistic Expectations

After you get your medical license, you'll be starting at the bottom. Remember that trust is earned. Don't expect to start your first day as an attending at the top of the totem pole. You'll need to earn the respect of your staff, colleagues, and patients. This will take time, but it will happen. As I said before, cultivate relationships.

Even if, when you were a resident, your attending expected you to know everything, don't believe for one minute that your attending knew it all either. When you become an attending, be okay with not having all the answers. Instead, recognize what you don't know, and seek help to find the answer.

Chapter 3 Summary

By the time a doctor completes medical school and residency, they may have spent a couple of decades dreaming about the day that they hold their own medical license in hand.

As you enter the field as a physician, keep these thoughts in mind:

- While it's easy to feel alone after you no longer have an attending by your side, tap into superiors in your reporting structure when you face challenges or have questions. Reporting structures should be in place to assist you, not smother or second-guess you.
- The "Oath" feels like an enormous responsibility—because it is! Doctors that try to do everything themselves will burn out quickly. Use your team to protect patient outcomes.
- Few doctors and even non-medical employees have bosses that teach self-care and empower their direct reports to take care

of themselves. If you don't prioritize your wellbeing, no one else will.

- Practice self-care, reminding yourself that you perform at your best level when you are rested, comfortable, and focused.

After so many years of training, some hold the identity of being a doctor so closely that they can experience an identity crisis if it is challenged, which is the topic of the following chapter.

Who Am I? The Identity Crisis

When a famous athlete or Hollywood celebrity has an identity crisis, we usually hear about it. For example, Miley Cyrus spoke openly about the identity crisis she suffered after she left her then-popular television show *Hannah Montana* (Tyagi 2021). Other celebrities feared losing their identities at the beginning of the COVID-19 pandemic and the ensuing shutdowns. One actress wondered about her "purpose" at the onset of lockdown, because she didn't know who she was outside of her career (Wenn 2021).

The same identity crises can occur in professional sports. In Randy Grimes's book, *Off Center,* former NFL center for the Tampa Bay Buccaneers described what he experienced when he went from being a known, recognized, and celebrated athlete during his playing days to becoming a *former* NFL player.

"Football had been my life since I was little," Randy said about his crisis of identity. "My dad was my first and favorite coach. Sunday morning, we worshipped God at church; Sunday afternoon and evening, we attended the church of the gridiron," he explained.

When asked about making his dream of being drafted into the NFL come true, his face looked much younger than his sixty-two years.

"Getting drafted by the Buccaneers felt like heaven on earth," he smiled broadly. "I mean, this club was going to pay me to play a game I'd have played for nothing. And the longer I played for the team, the more I enjoyed Tampa Bay. The fans loved me, even when our team didn't do well. They named the food court in the mall after me. As a local celebrity, I couldn't walk the street without having fans ask to take a picture with me."

And when asked about what changed when the new head coach gave him a pat on the shoulder and told him that his services wouldn't be needed any longer, he said, "No one prepared me for life after football. When I saw myself retiring from the game, I somehow imagined that I'd be the only guy still playing in his fifties, with gray hair and grandchildren," he said with a laugh. "It never dawned on me that I'd retire at thirty-two. I had no idea how to be anybody except a football player. I'd married my best friend and college sweetheart and had two beautiful children, but at first, my primary identity didn't come from being a husband or father. In my mind, I was a football player, and I couldn't see myself as having value outside the sport" (Grimes 2022).

It took Randy years before he confronted and conquered his identity crisis, but not until he first faced his addiction to prescription drugs that he started while still playing in the NFL.

While news articles and books like this focus on famous people who've struggled with their identities, identity crises can affect anyone. Physicians are particularly vulnerable.

Anyone can suffer from an identity when they go through a time of confusion and instability. This crisis is often characterized by questioning long-held values, relationships, self-worth, and purpose.

Younger people can experience this when they transition from childhood to adolescence or adolescence to adulthood. A *midlife crisis* is a type of identity crisis that is often associated with job/career change or loss, loss of vigor and perfect health, change in marital status, retirement, moving, death of parents, traumatic life event, or transitioning from being a parent to an "empty nester."

When someone is going through an identity crisis, they mourn for "the end of an era," leaving them with the belief that they have nothing to hold onto. Happiness, they believe, is behind them, and in front of them is nothing except uncertainty.

My Dad Longed to Change His Identity

From my father's perspective, his biological father, Glen Gregory, had abandoned him. But he hadn't. I later learned that Glen sent my father birthday cards every year, but Grandma Louise intercepted them. She wanted my father to have no contact with his own father. Then William R. Twombley came into my father's life, adopted my dad and his sister, and had another child; then he left too. By age eight, my dad lost two "father-figures," and neither explained or gave any reason for their departures.

As far as my dad knew, they left *because of him.*

When his mother traveled, she would drop him off to stay with his great uncle, a man my father loved, who served as the only permanent fixture in my dad's early years. My father wouldn't experience that connection again until he married my mother.

From all accounts I've heard about my father's early years, a few themes emerged. First, as I shared in Chapter 2, my dad excelled in school. Second, he frequently got into trouble, almost exclusively for drinking too much and then taking practical jokes "too far." Third, he somehow developed enough self-discipline to become an Eagle Scout, using the same tenacity that propelled him through medical school. Finally, my dad grew up with absolutely zero supervision, guidance, or parenting. No one ever placed rules on him, and he eventually raised himself. One family member shared with me that Daddy would come home, or not, as he chose. Since he did well in school, his mother didn't care what he did.

Clinical and developmental psychologist Diana Baumrind pioneered the idea that parenting styles fall into one of four groups.

1. *Authoritarian* parenting focuses on the rules, including obedience and punishment. Children raised by authoritarian parents often become great liars, because lying is how they learned to avoid punishment. These children may also develop anger issues and suffer from low self-esteem since their opinions didn't seem to matter at home.

2. *Authoritative* parents use positive discipline to pro-

actively prevent behavior problems. These parents use praise, encouragement, and rewards instead of overusing punishment to control their children's behaviors. Children raised by authoritative parents typically develop into responsible, successful adults capable of making good decisions and expressing their feelings.

3. *Permissive* parents live by the mantra "kids will be kids." They don't get actively involved in directing the behaviors or decisions of their children. When these parents make rules, they rarely follow through with consequences. Children raised by permissive parents often suffer from low self-esteem, unhappiness, and even health issues related to obesity, insufficient exercise, or dental cavities since they haven't been taught self-discipline.

4. *Neglectful* (or *uninvolved*) parents are uninvolved in nearly every aspect of their children's lives. Instead of checking on their child's physical and emotional well-being, they "check-out" of parenting. Children reared in neglectful environments often grow into the most unhappy adults with the lowest levels of self-esteem (Morin 2022).

I don't pretend to know Grandma Louise's motivation for remaining physically and emotionally detached from my father, but her neglectful parenting meant that my father never felt loved until he married my mother.

Randy Grimes loved the identity he found in playing professional football, but he had no idea what to do with life outside the gridiron. My father hated the identity he inherited from birth, so he sought a new one. After investing years of his life to become a doctor, he embraced that new identity fully. Unfortunately, he didn't identify himself as a father, parent, spouse, or friend. His identity began and ended with his profession. I shared that community members, patients, and even family members called my father Dr. T.

You might imagine that my father embraced the financial trappings that his medical degree eventually afforded him. However, he didn't pursue medicine to make more money, live in a fancy home, drive an expensive car, or take elaborate vacations. Dad became a doctor because he *loved* helping people, especially those without the means to help themselves. In fact, in lieu of family vacations, my dad took us on mission trips to Guatemala, something he did for thirty years.

Growing up with a shattered identity, my father entered a lifelong quest to build an identity that he could slip on like a pair of household slippers. But the problem with an identity that can be "put on" is that it can also wear out over time...and eventually get tossed out.

You Are More Than Your Highest Degree, Title, or Job

Fans of the 1960s television show *Star Trek* know the oft-repeated line by character Dr. Leonard McCoy on the U.S.S. Enterprise: "I'm a doctor, not a..." Whenever another character on the series asked Dr. McCoy to perform work outside of his area of expertise, he would say things like, "I'm a doctor, not an engineer," or "I'm a doctor, not a mechanic." Like the fictitious Dr. McCoy, my father never felt comfortable straying from the identity that his medical profession gave him.

Everyone worships something. As an increasing number of people in the US move away from traditional religion, the worship of work has taken its place in the form of *workism* (Thompson 2019). According to Derek Thompson of *The Atlantic,* workism is "the belief that work is not only necessary to economic production, but also the centerpiece of one's identity and life's purpose..."

Allowing work to become one's identity isn't new. The most common surname in the UK is Smith, which was derived from a person's profession as a locksmith, blacksmith, gunsmith, silversmith, and so on. "John the Smith" of the Middle Ages became "John Smith." Back then, occupations were considered something you inherited from your father or the adults working around you. If your dad was a blacksmith, you would likely become a blacksmith. If your dad was a carpenter, you would apprentice with him, learn the trade, and become a carpenter.

Education changed that. We no longer inherit or fall into jobs or careers. Instead, most of us get to choose the education that will prepare us for the work we wish to pursue. But that comes with a cost. According to Gallup, higher education corresponds with a greater likelihood a person will allow their work to become their identity. Seventy percent of American college graduates agree that they get their sense of identity from their job, whereas only 45 percent of Americans without a college degree affirm the same (Riffkin 2014).

Psychologist Anne Wilson said it this way: "If you tie [your self-worth] to your career, the successes and failures you experience will directly affect your self-worth. And because we live in a society where careers are less likely to be lifelong, if we switch or find ourselves out of a job, it can also become an identity crisis" (Morgan 2021).

Born into a home where his identity made him feel unseen, unloved, and unworthy, my father happily slipped into the role of doctor, something that made him feel seen, loved, and worthy. When my father's ability to continue serving as a doctor became threatened, he saw his identity disappearing before his eyes. He couldn't imagine not being the respected country doctor, especially when the events leading to his potential dismissal would have been a great embarrassment to him. I'll share more about this later.

Build an Identity in Which Being a Doctor Is But One Part

Jimmy Turner—an anesthesiologist, author, and host of *The Physician Philosopher* podcast—said it best: "Love your job. Be passionate about it. And be a really good doctor. But don't let it define you" (Turner 2022).

Invest in Personal Relationships

Let's assume that you're a doctor. How would you introduce yourself to someone you never met?

- Option 1: "My name is ____, and I've been a physician for eight years. I studied on the West Coast, but I did my residency in the Midwest before settling on the East Coast. I'm married with three children, and I love to hike and run in my free time."
- Option 2: "My name is ____. I live in New York

with my spouse of ten years and our three lovely children, two boys and a girl. I practice medicine at New York-Presbyterian Hospital. When I'm not at work or spending time with my family, you'll find me hiking or running."

When we're asked to introduce ourselves, what we say at the beginning of our introduction speaks to how we see ourselves. Those who use Option 1 are really saying, "This is the most important part of my identity." And it makes sense for several reasons. First, the path to becoming a physician is a journey of several years, more years than many marriages last. Second, as I shared earlier, people in the US, more so than people from other countries, tend to identify themselves with their professions. Finally, most family members are extremely proud of a loved one who reaches such a high achievement. Forty-five percent of the population that is married, and anyone with functioning reproductive organs, can produce offspring (Han 2022). Yet there are fewer than 100,000 general practitioners in the US, which is about 0.03 percent of the total population (Christensen 2023). Since attaining this high distinction is so rare, it makes sense that doctors would be proud of their credentials and want to mention them first.

However, prioritizing a profession over intimate, familial relationships can come at the expense of personal happiness. Happiness and even longevity are linked to our personal relationships (Mineo 2017). As radio host Bruce Williams famously cautioned, "Don't love anything that can't love you back."

I mentioned professional football player Randy Grimes earlier. Randy had played football since his childhood. He met his future wife, Lydia, at Baylor University, when they were both teenagers. The two married before he finished college, and then he got drafted by the Tampa Bay Buccaneers where he started and won accolades throughout his ten years in the National Football League. During his playing days, Randy had two children.

Even if Randy started playing football at birth, his football days lasted only thirty-two years. As of 2023, Randy and Lydia have been married for forty-one years. "Marrying Lydia was the best decision I've ever made," Randy told me. "Besides God, she's the most unchanging part of my life." Randy has now created an identity outside of football, attaching to the parts of his life that outlived his career. To weather the changes and stay connected to the crucial support of family, doctors should do the same.

My mother and father had a good marriage. But when I consider the amount of time my father invested in his work as opposed to his marriage and parenting, I know that being a doctor was his number one priority. And that took a toll—on himself and those around him. Whenever my father struggled with depression, my mother did her best to pull him back from the brink. It's common for married couples to vacillate between interdependent and codependent relationships. Interdependence happens when a couple feels intertwined yet operates autonomously, whereas codependency creates an unequal partnership where one person is elevated above the other. Part of me has wondered how much of my mother's own identity came from being married to a doctor, and how this may have affected her negatively. But she persisted.

Strong, healthy relationships can outlast jobs and careers.

Know What's Important to You

"If you were so financially set that you never needed to work another day of your life, where would you spend your time?" When researchers asked this question, nearly 35 percent of survey responders said that they would quit working, about 25 percent said they would work occasionally, and 25 said they would work part-time in a different field. Many people said that they would volunteer (Moore 2019).

Doctors might be the exception. Having spent more than thirty years of their lives learning and educating themselves prior to getting licensed to practice medicine, doctors will have spent as much time in school (if you include their entire history) as they will practice medicine if they retire at age sixty-five. It's hard to imagine investing that much of themselves into a job and career only to leave it behind and stay home. Obviously, doctors place a high value on education; or at the very least, they value what they can do with a higher education, like caring for patients.

I love my job as a pediatric nephrologist. When I'm not working, I often think about my patients and their families, because I truly care about them and their well-being. I treat each pediatric patient as if they were my own child. But make no mistake about it: if I learned that I had a short time to live, you wouldn't find me treating patients. Instead, I would spend time with my husband and children. Medically caring for others is my job, vocation, career, and calling. But loving my family is my highest value.

People suffering from an identity crisis often show one or more of these seven signs:

1. Having low self-esteem
2. Questioning their value or worth
3. Feeling lost or aimless
4. Lacking a sense of purpose or understanding their values
5. Feeling emotionally scattered (or having difficulty regulating their emotions)
6. Experiencing increased feelings of insecurity
7. Experiencing increased feelings of anxiety or depression

When someone experiences an identity crisis, they may latch onto whatever identity traits feel most positive. Since the symptoms of an identity crisis revolve around a sense of despair and hopelessness, it's not surprising that those struggling may adopt a façade of strength and security, almost to the point of seeming arrogant (think false bravado).

Look at the following list of values. If you don't see your top values listed, feel free to add them. This is not an exhaustive list. Circle the five values that you believe best represent you as a person or add your own. Be honest with yourself. Answer what you truly believe, not what you wish you could say is true for you. When you're done, review your top five choices and place a check mark next to your top three.

Achievement	Challenge	Faith	Humor	Optimism	Security
Adventure	Community	Fame	Influence	Pleasure	Service
Authenticity	Competency	Family	Justice	Popularity	Spirituality
Authority	Connection	Friendships	Kindness	Recognition	Stability
Autonomy	Contribution	Fun	Leadership	Religion	Success
Balance	Creativity	Growth	Learning	Reputation	Status
Beauty	Curiosity	Happiness	Love	Respect	Wealth
Boldness	Determination	Harmony	Loyalty	Responsibility	Wisdom
Compassion	Fairness	Honesty	Openness	Safety	Work

Write your top three values in the lines provided:

1. ____

2. ____

3. ____

Let's say that your top three values are family, kindness, and love. It should follow that you would spend much of your time in activities involving family, creating kindness, and sharing love. Friend and leadership speaker Scott Carbonara says it this way: "If you want to know where someone's heart is, look at where their feet are pointing."

Now let me ask you: what would you do if you had a week to live? If you don't like your answer, I have good news for you. It's not too late to change how you live your life and where you spend your time.

People may live outside of their values, but it comes at the price of happiness. A doctor named Danielle left the profession when she found her work as a doctor created conflict with her values. "I was not the person, wife, or mother I wanted to be," she shared. "I spent my days in a constant state of rush, rush, rush, never smelling the proverbial roses. I never had time to do anything for myself and could barely manage to provide basic care for my daughter. As for being a wife, I was just a moody cow most days" (Fork 2020).

The mattress companies suggest you buy the best mattress you can afford, since you spend a third of your life sleeping. (Although if you spend a third of your life sleeping, you're probably not a doctor.) We sleep because we need to recharge our bodies, not because sleeping releases pleasure. We spend another third of our lives working, so I certainly believe we should find a vocation that brings us meaning and joy. But the final third of our lives we have for ourselves. How much of our lives can we live out of sync with our values before we feel conflicted?

Set Boundaries Around Your Values

When you think of a wealthy neighborhood, you probably picture a gated community and homes with security systems. People with fine, valuable possessions protect their belongings. *Why should we be less protective of our values than of the things we own?*

Once my father adopted the doctor identity, he set that as his top priority. Everything else fit around that value. Jesus Christ said, "No man can serve two masters." The same holds true for our values. One of our values will always come out on top. If you value free time, you'll have to say no to picking up every extra work shift available. If you value financial security, you can't keep plunging into crippling financial debt. If you value your family, you won't likely spend time away from them voluntarily.

Yes, duties often conflict. If we love our family, we can't simply declare that they are our number one priority without providing for their needs. But we can safeguard our time with them even while working a demanding job.

Evaluate how you live your values today. Do you regularly feel guilty for how you spend your time? Do you feel that one part of your life claims more of your attention and time than you would like? Do you have conflict with people in your life about your inability to "show up" and be present? If so, realign the finite hours in your day so you protect the things that matter most to you.

Chapter 4 Summary

Criminal defense attorney and professor Bryan Stevenson said, "Everyone is more than the worst thing they've ever done." While that's true, it's very easy to fall into the belief that we're *as valuable as the highest level we've ever achieved*. Whether you're a former professional athlete or a physician, you might connect your entire identity to your best play or your highest degree, which can lead to an identity crisis.

A way to prevent having your entire identity linked to your profession is to strive to balance the various buckets of your life. Yes, work is a part of who you are. But you are also a part of your family, personal relationships, friendships, community, and so on. If you root all components of your life to your values, you will never lose sight of what is most important to you.

In the following chapter, I'll explain more about what happens to many doctors who fail to create an identity outside of their profession.

Burnout and the Missing Off Switch

The Organization for Economic Co-operation and Development (OECD) is comprised of representatives from thirty-eight democracies with market-based economies that create policy standards for sustained economic growth. Did you know that of those thirty-eight countries, only four don't adhere to a maximum work week? The US is one of those countries (Miller 2023).

Think about how many hours you spend each week thinking or talking about work and office-related projects outside of work. Besides US employees working longer hours each week than worked in most other countries, most workers use technologies to stay connected 24/7. Regardless of someone's profession, many employees feel obligated to stay connected to work outside of "normal business hours." Perhaps that's why full-time employees with a minimum of a bachelor's degree spend, on average, 8.25 hours at work each weekday and 4.35 hours each weekend day continuing to work (US Dept. of Labor 2023)!

This especially holds true in the medical field, where some of the work involves life and death decisions. *Did I remember to log all client records? Did I make the right diagnosis? Did I prescribe the best medicine? Have I logged onto the portal to answer my patient's medical questions?* It's no wonder that many people working in medicine come home at the end of their shifts, but their minds are elsewhere.

The term *hyper focus* is defined as "a phenomenon that reflects one's complete absorption in a task, to a point where a person appears to completely ignore or 'tune out' everything else." Clinical research often uses that word in connection with ADHD, autism, and schizophrenia.

Psychologist Mihaly Csikszentmihalyi coined another word that's closely related to hyper focus called *flow*. He described flow as having eight characteristics:

1. Complete concentration on the task
2. Clarity of goals and rewards in mind, along with immediate feedback
3. Transformation of time (speeding up/slowing down)
4. The experience is intrinsically rewarding
5. Effortlessness and ease
6. There is a balance between challenge and skills
7. Actions and awareness are merged, losing self-conscious rumination
8. There is a feeling of control over the task

I've often wondered if, after years of school, residency, and completing medical boards, doctors may slip into a hyper focus or flow mode as a default habit that stays with them even after completing their education. That might help explain why so many medical professionals struggle to switch off the topic of medicine to engage in other activities.

My Father Never Stopped Working

My dad was a workaholic. When Dad wasn't working at his clinic or in the emergency room, or doing rounds at the hospital, he saw patients at home. When we lived in a small town, people would sometimes just show up at our door after hours for treatment. I remember my dad stitching someone up at the kitchen table more than once.

As a child, my father once took me on a daddy-daughter trip to Disney World. But looking back on that trip now as an adult, I see it as another sign that my father couldn't stop thinking about work. What brought us to Orlando for that Disney trip? My father attended a medical conference. He spent the day at the conference, and then he walked around Disney with me in his leftover time. He loved me and wanted to spend time with me. He still managed to make the trip special for me. But that trip would never have happened were it not tied to his work as a doctor.

More than Dad working all the time, as I've suggested, he struggled to form emotional bonds with those around him. Until he met and married my mother, he had no close friends. My father loved his family. None of us doubted that. Dad came home, but he never really connected with his family.

Usually, he responded to a hug from family members by leaving his arms down at his sides. When he did hug, he practiced the side-hug, the kind you give to someone you don't feel comfortable touching. My father grew up without physical affection, so it's not surprising that he didn't know how to show it to others. He never initiated saying the words, "I love you." Instead, if we said, "I love you," he would say, "Love you too." He was never at ease with sharing positive emotions or affection with us. Even in his final letter to me, he did not write, "I love you."

In his book *Pudd'nhead Wilson*, Mark Twain wrote, "The wise man saith, 'Put all your eggs in the one basket and WATCH THAT BASKET'" (Twain 2005).

The basket in which my father placed all his eggs was labeled "medical doctor." Whether he worked in the clinic or in his head at home, his heart and mind stayed in medicine. What was my father thinking about at home? Doctoring.

While I haven't seen statistics, I imagine that most doctors take their work home with them at a level that's higher than other college graduates. We all have a reticular activating system (RAS), a bundle of neurons at the base of the spinal column that's about the size of a little finger. While it's small, this part of the brain serves as the gatekeeper for all information that our brain receives (Thome et al. 2019, 1–14). Neurologists tell us that the human brain can process eleven million bits of information every second, which is far more than our conscious mind can sift through. The RAS pairs down those millions of pieces of information to the forty to fifty most relevant and useful bits (Agarwal 2020).

The nature of the work that doctors perform means that the forty to fifty bits of information that reach their consciousness at any given second involve sickness, injury, treatment, medication, and diagnoses. Doctors can easily become singularly focused to the point of obsessing about patient outcomes 24/7. No matter where they go or what they're doing, many struggle switching off from being a doctor.

Doctors know that patients get sick on holidays, weekends, and after hours. That's the nature of the job. Once a doctor has a family, every minute gets filled with work and family, leaving little time for outside interests and hobbies or even alone time.

My father eventually developed some interests outside of medicine, some of which would prove healthier than others. Some people with disposable income collect fine wines, art, and high-end cars. My dad had no use for those things. Instead, he began an eclectic collection of assorted junk, like Christmas Seals, the little stamps placed on mail around the holidays to raise awareness for diseases of the lungs, air pollution, and influenza. He had full sheets of Christmas Seals from every year they were ever made. He also got interested in Civil War relics and started collecting Confederate money, which eventually led him to save currency from all the places he traveled during his medical mission trips.

Somewhere along the way, Dad started collecting pocketknives. None of his knives were expensive or rare; he would just pick up the kind you see at a local hardware store. By the time he died, he had hundreds of knives in his collection.

Then he started collecting firearms. He had always been fascinated with antique guns. Living in the country most of his life, Dad viewed guns as a way of life. We lived on a swamp in the country, and there were no houses within shooting range, so our backyard turned into a gun range. Even the local law enforcement officers would shoot at our range. My dad eventually got his Federal Firearms License (FFL), which is a gun dealer's license. Local police, politicians, and farmers all bought guns from him.

Over time, he assembled an arsenal, and we had guns in every corner of the house. There was likely not a legal gun made that he didn't have at our house at one time or another. When he had our house built, he placed a full-size gun safe in the house prior to the roof being installed (the safe was too big to fit through standard-sized doors). I didn't find this at all odd, maybe because this was the norm I grew up with.

Our backyard abutted Bear Swamp, a place teeming with wild animals. Guns became a tool to keep us safe in the wilderness around us. We had nothing but farmland and woods between our house and the nearest town, and the road had minimal streetlights. Worried about my safety if my car broke down, my father gave me a gun and a cell phone (one of the original, large, mobile box phones) to keep in the car. Once again, it never even dawned on me that this was atypical.

As our country continues to debate the Second Amendment, I can understand how some readers might wonder why I never thought twice about having a gun in my car and guns in every room in the house while growing up. Those growing up in large cities like Chicago or Los Angeles might associate guns with drugs, gangs, violence, and drive-by shootings. But growing up in the country, guns were an extension of a person's hand. By the time I turned five years old, my great, great aunt Alice had taught me how to load and shoot an old, single-shot .22 rifle. I loved that gun when I was a kid and looked forward to shooting it every time we visited her. When she died, she left me that gun, and I still have it to this day. It's one of my truly cherished items. I grew up around guns and developed a great respect for them.

Once Dad finished having the house constructed, he built a shop out in the woods which gave him more privacy. He didn't actually build it; instead, he had some old houses and barns moved out into the woods, and he converted them into his shops. One of the shops became his "man cave," while the others became storage units. He would tinker with his guns in his shop, learning how to make home-made silencers for them so that he wouldn't scare the dogs with his shooting. The shop became his second home, the place where he could isolate and spend time in his head.

Having a special place to decompress is a healthy habit for most people, and it was for my dad. At first. But it didn't stay healthy. He started smoking and drinking in his man cave. Since he was out of sight, no one knew the full extent of his addictions. His struggling mental health and drinking problems, coupled with his history of risky behaviors and easy access to multiple firearms, gave him limit-less opportunities to act impulsively.

Why Doctors Lack an Off Switch

The fault for busyness doesn't lie solely with the physicians. The medical system has created and allowed this structure. As I've shared, even when a doctor is off, they're sent emails and expected to answer. When they try to take off, they return to work with inboxes full of patient questions, labs to review, and notes to write, not to mention the hundreds of emails waiting to be answered. Doctors who manage to take a week off get punished with double workloads once they return. It's no wonder that a physician cannot shut their mind off even on vacation.

Another issue in the medical system that contributes to this increased workload is electronic medical records (EMRs). While EMRs have some great features, documenting time has increased exponentially since its inception (more on this later).

Another huge issue is insurance company payment requirements, as I've touched on in earlier chapters. Insurance companies require a lot of extra documentation for you to bill for your time (again, more on this later). Insurance companies want information that isn't always necessary to take care of a patient. But since they set the rules on what they will pay and how doctors must perform to get paid, physicians end up jumping through a lot of extra hoops to please them, and this takes time. Doctors spend a lot of nights and weekends documenting in the EMR, and it's expected that they will do this. Hospitals offer EMR optimization, but the documentation still takes more time than it did in pre-EMR days. Now hospitals are requiring you to have your notes done in 30 days. If you do not, they take the potential revenue that the system would have collected from this patient encounter out of your salary! If you think the physician shortage is bad now, can you imagine how this punitive measure will make it better?

Prior authorizations are another issue. Some medications require prior authorization, because they are extremely expensive. It takes a lot of time to do this paperwork. While doctors get some help from their office staff, a lot of the work doctors do require a "peer-to-peer" call to get a medication approved for a patient. This is non-billable time.

Creating a Life Outside of Scrubs

I have a colleague who once a year does a "staycation" in her own town. She rents a hotel in downtown Charleston and leaves her kids at home with her husband. She goes out to dinner, a show, drinks, or whatever she wants. Sometimes she goes alone, sometimes she takes a girlfriend.

> When I go to a conference, I try to take a half day to a who day to recharge. I sleep late, get a massage, read a book by the pool, etc.
>
> The point is that you have to have a life outside of work.

Researchers began a Harvard men's study on happiness in 1938. (If you're wondering why Harvard choose to study men only, it was because Harvard didn't accept women at the time.) Gathering health records from more than seven hundred people every two years, they sent survey participants detailed questions about their lives.

One participant who had served as a physician for nearly fifty years reported what he missed most about work. His answer is telling: "Absolutely nothing about the work itself. I miss the people and the friendships." The summary after eighty-plus years of research gives us an invaluable guide to creating happiness at work and into retirement: invest in relationships now (Shulz and Waldinger 2023). Don't assume you'll just naturally make new friends once you retire.

While it's important to find hobbies to recharge our batteries, we also need to surround ourselves with people who give our lives meaning and purpose. If you struggle to make friendships today, you will probably have just as much difficulty once you quit working.

Thinking back to my father, he never developed deep, intimate relationships outside of my mom and his children. Of course, he had friends who he could drink a beer and talk about superficial things with, but that was the extent of his relationships. Instead of talking to friends when he felt troubled, he held his struggles inside and isolated himself. One study found that isolation and loneliness carry the same health risk as smoking fifteen cigarettes a day (Kroll 2022).

Healthcare professionals know of the research showing what happens to individuals who lack strong social connections. People lacking in social connections have health risks including:

- Greater risk for depression and anxiety
- Elevated levels of stress and inflammation, coronary artery disease, gut dysfunction, abnormal insulin regulation, problems with the immune system, and cancer
- Cognitive and functional decline, including dementia
- Decreased immune response to infection
- Slower recovery from injury, surgery, and illness
- Premature death (50 percent increased risk) (HCBH 2021)

In all my years of school, I never took a class—or spent a portion of a class—learning how to build relationships or develop social connections. Given that medical school is designed to teach students to identify and treat illness, it's no wonder why there are no required classes on topics like personal finance, friendships, or happiness. Yet who better than doctors to know the effects that out-of-control stress, loneliness, and sorrow have on the body? Sadly, not all physicians practice healthy habits and hobbies in their personal lives.

Developing a Balanced Life

The proverb says, "All work and no play makes Jack a dull boy." I shared earlier that most working professionals have a maximum of eight hours each day to recharge away from work. Time spent outside of work and engaging in rest gives us the opportunity to spend with friends and family. In addition to spending time with others, this is the block of time where we can invest in outside interests such as hobbies.

Some time ago, I read that people should make time for three hobbies: one for physical fitness, one for creative enjoyment, and one for making money. During my years as a medical professional, I've known colleagues that used their downtime to run or hike, collect things like cars or antiques, and take up hobby-farming or breeding animals like dogs. The possibilities are endless.

I recharge with my family and pets. I have a "little zoo" at my house, because animals make me happy. We have a banana ball python (Loki), three sugar gliders (Roe, Boba, Crabby), and two dogs (Mae-sadly she passed before book was published- and Ginger) inside the house and six koi, two goldfish, and various other pond creatures in our backyard pond. We will also have Finnigan (Frankie's service dog), who will join us in the summer of 2024. I also take time to garden, growing everything from tomatoes and peppers to turmeric and ginger. I enjoy fermenting my own hot sauces with fruits and vegetables from my backyard. And I dabble (a very small amount) in stocks and cryptocurrency.

By taking time away from work to recharge, I have the focus and energy to dedicate to my patients and administrative duties when I'm back at work. When my life becomes hectic and I don't get downtime, my work, sleep, and relationships suffer.

Most of us start to develop our interests and hobbies during childhood. A friend of mine is an avid gardener, something he learned from his father. While he hated everything to do with flowers, trees, vegetables, and landscaping as his dad's unpaid, unwilling apprentice, my friend started to understand the joy of creating beauty from the ground when he grew older.

The same is true with appreciating music, cooking, baking, running, rock collecting, traveling, and other hobbies. When a parent takes an interest in something and exposes their children to it in a positive way, the children have a good chance of growing up to love the same activities.

My father loved music. I still have all of his old vinyl albums and his antique record player. It makes me happy to see them and even listen to them occasionally. We went to concerts together to hear artists such as Hank Williams Jr., The Marshall Tucker Band, The Charlie Daniels Band, and The Allman Brothers Band. My father instilled his love of music in me from a very young age. I hated learning the piano as a child, and now wish I could play better. He encouraged me to sing and play the saxophone which I did for years! I was even offered a full scholarship to college for voice to an out of state small college that I turned down because I wanted to go to medical school in state. Music was and is when I feel closest to my father.

While my father developed some good hobbies later in life, once again, he had no positive role model in his childhood home to be exposed to healthy hobbies. Instead of doing something sustainable and good for his health, he let his at-risk behaviors become his way of letting off steam.

Plenty of hobbies are low cost or come with a small startup cost. Keeping in mind the three hobbies that everyone should have, what can you do for your health, your creativity, and your pocketbook?

Invest in a Hobby of Physical Fitness

For the price of basic equipment like running or hiking shoes, a racquet, a bicycle, or gardening tools, you can get healthy physical activity that stretches and tones your muscles, reduces your blood pressure and cholesterol levels, burns fat, balances your blood sugar, and reduces feelings of stress.

Here are some hobbies that could jump-start your physical fitness:

Walking	Weight Training	Pickleball
Running	Jumping Rope	Rollerblading
Hiking	Basketball	Skateboarding
Skiing	Tennis	Swimming
Kayaking or Canoeing	Surfing	Frisbee
Biking	Dancing	Gardening
Soccer	Volleyball	Softball
Martial Arts	Curling	Ice Skating
Bowling	Hockey	Football
Gardening	Kite Flying	Waterskiing
Rugby	Yoga	Horseback Riding

Many people like to enjoy these hobbies with a friend, which can also help in creating key social connections—thereby building another important pillar in your health. It can also be easier to get into a sport, or sustain it, if you don't do it alone. A runner friend told me about how much more quickly the time passes on her long training runs if she brings along a friend to chat with, for example. Others like these activities for the alone time they offer, which is perfectly fine and healthy too.

Invest in a Hobby that Inspires Your Creativity

Creative hobbies also include activities you can do alone or with others. Even something like collecting can be a creative hobby when it involves hunting for a unique item to add to your collection. Creative hobbies have been shown to stimulate brain function, reduce cognitive decline, improve mental health, and increase your ability to learn new skills.

Here are some hobbies that could serve as creative outlets:

Photography	Painting/Drawing	Digital or Graphic Arts
Writing	Crocheting or Knitting	Woodworking
Dancing	Landscaping	Collecting
Reading	Singing	Sculpting
Scrapbooking	Acting	Board Games

A friend of mine spent a weekend cleaning out the garage of the home he had recently purchased. He found old bicycle parts, sheets of scrap metal, and cans of spray paint. Instead of taking these items to the dump, he cut the sheet metal into fin shapes before painting them bright colors. Then he fastened the fins to the outer edge of the metal bicycle wheels. Using tall metal poles and the forks of bikes, he created whirligigs that he used to decorate his yard. Before long, friends and neighbors asked him to make them whirligigs, creating a pastime that gave him a perfect, inexpensive creative outlet.

Invest in Hobbies That Can Increase the Size of Your Pocketbook

Some hobbies can make you money. Years ago, a friend of mine got interested in identifying and foraging for wild mushrooms. As he continued to learn, he started inoculating hardwood logs with the mycelia from edible mushrooms like lion's mane, shitake, and oyster mushrooms. Before long, he had more edible mushrooms than he could eat, so he started selling them at a local farmer's market. Not only did he earn some extra money, but he also made new friends each weekend. Hobbies that can turn a profit can improve one's understanding of how to run a business, since they require rudimentary skills like negotiating, marketing, conducting a cost-benefit analysis, and so on.

Here are some hobbies that can turn a profit:

Collecting	Gardening	Farming
Restoring Antiques	Raising Chickens	Making Birdhouses
Painting	Photography	Website Design
Stained glass	House Flipping	Freelance Writing
Tutoring or Teaching	Professional Development	Coaching

Your Action Plan

Just like we don't develop relationships automatically, we don't always find healthy, positive hobbies without some effort. Write down at least three hobbies that you currently practice or are willing to start, including at least one in each of these categories:

Physical Fitness	Creativity	Potential Money-Makers
_____________	_____________	_____________
_____________	_____________	_____________
_____________	_____________	_____________

Next, evaluate your level of satisfaction with the depth of your social relationships and connections. Having a larger number of connections doesn't necessarily lead to greater satisfaction; rather, it's the closeness you feel to those who are in your life that matters. For example, introverts might have a small handful of friends and close confidants, while extroverts might have dozens. Think about the *warmth* of those relationships, not the raw number.

In the table that follows, circle the number that most accurately represents your current satisfaction level with the *depth and warmth* of your social relationships and connections.

After completing this table, answer the following questions:

Strongly dissatisfied	Dissatisfied	Slightly dissatisfied	Neither satisfied nor dissatisfied	Slightly satisfied	Satisfied	Strongly satisfied
1	2	3	4	5	6	7

1. What investments do you actively make to keep those in your immediate circle of intimacy (family members and close friends) close?
2. What investments can you make to expand your circle of intimacy to include colleagues and acquaintances?
3. How can you further expand your circle of intimacy to build relationships with people like neighbors and those you cross paths with periodically?

Chapter 5 Summary

Workers, especially in the US, tend to work long hours, and some even seem to link how hard they work with their self-esteem. *I work hard, so I must be valuable,* they reason. Perhaps no industry buys into this idea more than healthcare, which tends to silently communicate to its workers, *If you aren't tired all of the time, you aren't working hard enough.*

It's time for physicians to embrace the "work hard, play hard" philosophy. When we lack activities that we're enthusiastic about and love engaging in, we just end up working more. Or thinking about work, which is often equally stressful.

Balance your priorities and rest your working brain by identifying and spending time in hobbies that allow you to recharge.

Next, I will expand on the challenges that envelop doctors while they toil in their roles daily until retirement.

Early Career Through Retirement

In 1944, President Franklin Delano Roosevelt chose Harry Truman as his vice-presidential running mate—a role Truman would serve in for eighty-two days before FDR's sudden death on April 12, 1945, catapulted Truman into the "accidental" presidency. During those eighty-two days, Truman only met with Roosevelt twice. Truman never took part in a single intelligence briefing, even though the US fought in two theaters of war, one in Europe and another in the Pacific. Truman never met with any world leaders, and he wasn't privy to the details of the Manhattan Project, the top-secret mission to develop a viable nuclear bomb (Cohen 2020).

Truman would serve the rest of FDR's term as President of the United States while the war in the Pacific reached its height. Without even having met with Winston Churchill or Joseph Stalin, Truman worked with his peers in the Allied powers to broker the end of the war in Europe. Then he turned his attention to the war in the Pacific where he made what is often considered the toughest decision any world leader has ever faced: the use of nuclear weapons to break the will of the enemy. After the war, Truman led the country during the onset of the Cold War, pioneering both the Truman Doctrine and NATO. Truman's leadership was instrumental in the Berlin Airlift and Marshall Plan as well as the United States's involvement in Korea to repel the Soviet-backed invasion by North Korea.

You're probably wondering why I inserted a short history lesson about the thirty-third President of the United States in a book about physician mental health and suicide. Here's why: once doctors finish residency, the training wheels come off. They are prepared for many medical situations that surface, but they will face many challenges that they had never anticipated. Just as Truman made decisions that ushered the world into a new nuclear age, doctors will face decades of new challenges on a regular basis. And they'll need to figure it out as they go.

Debt Meets the Spending Trap

The first challenge many new doctors face is with their personal finances, as I've hinted at earlier in this book. Fortunately, my father never spent beyond his means or fell into the spending trap. In fact, no one seeing my dad in his truck or meeting him on the street would guess he was a doctor. He didn't dress or act the part in his lifestyle. He lived modestly.

Yet I've known many doctors who, after spending years preparing to become a doctor and accruing six-figure student debt, grow hungry to exchange their ramen noodle diet for caviar. These doctors start accruing new, enormous debt because of oversized spending habits that will deliver them constant financial pressure.

Dr. Sanjiv Lakhia explains the lifestyle creep that often

accompanies the *rags to riches* phenomenon that physicians can experience:

Many physicians literally jump into the "1 percent" income bracket overnight, transitioning from a resident's salary to that of a practicing clinician....Society holds physicians up to a certain wealth standard and expectation that can be unrealistic to maintain. If not careful, physicians can quickly find themselves living a glamorous, expensive lifestyle. Stress can quickly mount to meet very high production standards at work in efforts to maintain a standard of living that is hard to pull back from (Tenny 2020).

As I shared earlier, the average medical school graduate amasses more than $250,000 in student loan debt. Yet the average annual salary for a medical doctor is $294,000 (Nomad Health 2018). *So why do some doctors struggle financially?*

To answer that question, consider lottery winners. Winning a $2 billion jackpot would change anyone's life. But were that lottery winner to take the lump sum payment, they would end up with $929 million. After paying federal taxes of about $344 million, they would end up with $585 million. And if they were to live in a state with income tax, those winnings would drop further. After the government takes its portion, the winner would still have a huge chunk of money—unless and until they make multiple large purchases. Then they would get hit again with sales tax—especially on the luxury items that many lottery winners splurge on. Of course, friends and family members they have never met also might come out of nowhere to ask for handouts, loans, or "investment opportunities" in their new businesses.

There are two things that medical doctors and lottery winners have in common. First, their take-home pay (net) is significantly smaller than the gross dollar amount they earn. Second, most doctors inherently have the same amount of money management skills as lottery winners, meaning none. In case you're wondering how things work out for lottery winners, approximately one-third of large jackpot winners end up bankrupt (Zagorsky 2022).

While medical professionals aren't as likely as lottery winners to declare bankruptcy, financial stress takes its toll in several ways. Half of all medical doctors report feeling burned out. Financial stress is the second leading cause of physician depression. And physicians have the highest suicide rate of any profession (Tenny 2020).

Few physicians know how to manage their money, much less how to transition successfully when they go from "rags to riches." Of course, their lack of money management skills isn't because they lack intelligence; rather, they've applied their intelligence and years of study to learn how to care for patients instead of mastering how to invest wisely.

New doctors will face the temptation to spend instead of save, or they may save only in only one asset, such as the stock market. My father lost a lot of his savings in the Great Recission of 2007. This was a huge stressor to him, and per his own words, was likely one of the contributing factors to his eventual death. I'll explain more later.

Doctors who don't practice sound money-management will often find themselves being owned by the high-paying jobs that they can't afford to leave.

Business 101 Is Required

When Dad first opened his practice, he had no experience running a small business, nor did he possess the financial acumen required to "keep the lights on." Medical school prepared him to manage patients, but not to manage his money or business.

Dad wanted to practice medicine so he could positively impact the health and lives of his patients. He never wanted to run a business, lead a team, become the "boss," or serve as an administrator. Yet he got pressed into these positions by default.

As a permanent fixture in a small-town hospital, he knew more about what needed to be done than anyone else in the area. All the staff looked to him for solutions. Always wanting to please others, Dad felt like he couldn't refuse to assume administrative responsibility.

Dad's "promotions" meant he could delegate responsibility to others. Yet always wishing to please others, he rarely did. Instead of finding another doctor or advanced practice provider to fill a shift, he worked it himself. When equipment broke or supplies ran out, my dad had to find a solution. Because of Dad's lack of leadership training, he believed that he as the leader must do more than anyone else in the clinic or hospital.

Not surprisingly, Dad hated every minute of this part of his role. Not only did he lack training in personal finance and self-care, but he also didn't know how to run a business or work within the healthcare matrix. When something broke, he asked for a replacement. When things got busy, he asked for more staffing. But those requests would fall on deaf ears, since he didn't submit his requests with accompanying proformas, cost benefit analyses, and so on. My father didn't know those things were required, and even if he had, he didn't know how to execute them.

The week my dad died, he tried to get a specialist to come to the ER to see a patient, and the specialist refused. This stressed my father more than anyone could have imagined. He felt that taking care of patients was no longer the healthcare system's priority. Why would a fellow physician refuse to come see a patient? He felt that the actions of this physician represented the entire healthcare system, and there was nothing he could do about it.

Today, physicians serve in many different healthcare roles. After earning medical degrees, completing residency, and serving as doctors for a short time, some go on to get a master's in business administration (MBA), master's of public health, or master's of healthcare administration degree to receive specific leadership training in the healthcare industry. These doctors typically don't typically end up remaining in frontline medicine or middle management positions, such as a medical director or division chief. Instead, their career goals are higher up the chain, such as CEO, chief medical officer, or president of a hospital system.

But when my dad entered healthcare, doctors were never encouraged to learn how to run a business or contribute to its bottom line. Doctors saw patients. Yet the more time a doctor worked in direct care, the more likely that doctor would be asked to assume administrative responsibilities, regardless of their aptitude or desire to serve in such a role.

In 1969, Laurence J. Peter and Raymond Hull wrote *The Peter Principle,* a book outlining the concept of how people in organizations often rise through the ranks due to their competence in one discipline. Sadly, the skills they used in earlier positions to achieve high results don't translate into success in their new roles.

In healthcare, this historically led to the best doctor or surgeon getting promoted to administrative jobs that had less to do with direct patient care than with making business decisions and leading others—as well as filling out paperwork and signing forms.

In my own experience, I stepped into the role of division director because the former one quit and moved away. With no training, schooling, or mentoring, I had to learn the role while working the job, which is not the most effective instructional model. Like my father, I never wanted to do anything except direct patient care. Through trial and error, I got the job done, but needless stress was put on me and those around me while I learned the role. Along the way, the hospital discovered that I had an aptitude for the administrative role, and I was given additional leadership responsibilities. However, that was not my intended career path. However much I do enjoy it now, it was not an easy role.

Doctors opting to work in private practice must know business basics if they're going to run a smooth operation; if they work in a hospital system, they must learn how their employer runs their business. Business acumen isn't a *nice-to-have* skill. Doctors who don't know how to manage the business side of practicing medicine run the risk of: cheating themselves out of money they've earned for their services, running into trouble with their employer for failing to manage their resources appropriately, or being taken advantage of by their employer by not being adequately compensated for their work.

This next statement may sound like an attack on men, but it's not. And I'm going to say it even if it raises a few eyebrows. Hospital leaders include two groups: White males and everyone else. Females and underrepresented minority physicians are rarely given the opportunity, whether qualified or not, to assume any significant leadership role unless an organization is actively working to improve the diversity of their leadership team.

Let me use academic medical centers (AMCs) as one example. Currently, females make up less than thirty percent of medical professionals serving in full professor roles, and only twenty-two percent of center directors, division chiefs, department chairs, and deans, are women (Chaudron et all, 2023). While males fill most of leadership roles. Globally, women make up nearly seventy percent of health and social care workers and almost ninety percent of nurses and midwifes; however, only around twenty-five percent of females working in healthcare are selected for leadership roles.

Secretary-General of the United Nations, Antonio Guterres, said it best: "It is time to stop trying to change women [and other underrepresented groups], and start changing the systems that prevent them from achieving their potential" (Closing the Leadership Gap, 2021).

I believe that health systems need to attract and retain leaders that reflect the demographic of the patients they serve. White males are not the only group that visits the doctor. In fact, White males are less likely to seek medical care than same-aged females. Successful healthcare systems of the future will prioritize increasing diversity in both the doctor's and executive's offices.

The Hippocratic Oath Meets the Healthcare Matrix

My dad envisioned a job where he would go in, treat patients, get paid, and go home. Imagine his surprise when, after spending the first thirty-plus years of his life preparing to practice medicine, he discovered that a disproportionate amount of "patient care" involved coding, charting, and billing—processes that had nothing to do with treating patients and everything to do with getting paid. And even then, he wasn't guaranteed that he could treat patients in the way he thought was best.

The Healthcare Matrix Directs Patient Care, Not the Physician

Hospital systems keep tightening the strings on budgets to the point where—despite having published values or marketing materials to the contrary—patient care seems like an afterthought. Administrators appear to make decisions with little consideration of how their policies impact patients. Rather, their concern is how the decisions they make affect their bottom line (money). When these healthcare decisions are made by those furthest removed from the patients (who doctors are meant to serve), problems arise.

I'm not suggesting that money doesn't matter; of course, leaders must balance a budget and consider what can and can't be afforded within a practice or system. They also must manage compliance and changing regulations. But those decisions must be balanced with the bedside implications—for providers and their patients—of any change.

Changes in the healthcare industry, just like the tech sector, evolve quickly, and the people making these decisions are often out of touch with practicing medicine. Many hospital administrators haven't treated patients or practiced medicine on the front line for twenty years. Yet those administrators make decisions that directly impact those actually performing the patient care, and their choices are often based on their outdated experience and expertise. As hospital systems expand, systems will regularly change, and policies will often get created and implemented without consulting with working physicians; this can cause doctors to believe that *the needs of the system outweigh the needs of the patient.*

To add injury to insult, at the end of a long shift, doctors return to their computers to catch up on email, where they find a message from hospital administration saying something like, "I'm sure you feel a sense of pride working for a hospital system that takes great care in our patient-centric decision-making." When administrators blast these yay-rah-rah emails to their employees, doctors quickly decipher the coded language: "improved patient care" means "saving and/or making the hospital system more money."

Is it any wonder that healthcare professionals can become jaded?

Not satisfied with micromanaging the work that doctors perform, hospital administrators also have embraced the concept of *relative value units* (RVUs), a process where doctors must document and put a price tag on every task throughout the day. By implementing RVUs, physicians who'd avoided experiencing a crisis of identity up to this point are then told, "Here's the value of your individual contribution today."

Historically, older doctors make more money while doing less "work." This is because RVUs don't place a value on their work in mentoring newer physicians. Instead, RVUs put a dollar figure on each *clinical activity* a doctor performs, prompting experienced doctors to spend less time mentoring. To "justify your salary," higher paid, experienced doctors can do one of two things: enter administration where they are removed from direct patient care or see more patients.

When you see an older doctor performing five or six surgeries each day, you might be comforted to know that they have decades of experience. At the same time, a high-paid eighty-year-old doctor working in direct care must carry the same workload as someone half that age. Few institutions pay for experience. Instead, they pay for doctors to serve as administrators, and for productivity (seeing a large number of patients each day).

Aa a state record-holder in cross-country and track and field her freshman year in high school, Brooke's running future ended when hip pain made her unable to walk without extreme discomfort. After four unsuccessful surgeries to correct her problem failed to provide relief, she met with a seasoned, world-renowned surgeon at one of the top-rated hospitals in the country. After reviewing her medical records and meeting with her, he told her that she needed a femoral derotational osteotomy to correct femoral torsion, a procedure that corrects a femur that turns too far to the inside of the body.

It's not an easy operation. The surgeon cuts and breaks the femoral bone and then rotates it so many degrees to correct its position. In Brooke's case, she needed both legs done, which meant two surgeries. After the cut and break, her femurs would be rotated in an outward direction fifteen degrees before a metal rod would be placed inside each bone to add strength as they healed.

On the early morning of the first of these surgeries, as an eighteen-year-old "adult," Brooke wasn't allowed to bring a family member with her due to the COVID pandemic. So, when the surgeon came to see her in pre-op—for what most patients would assume is a routine visit before entering the operating room—she dialed her dad to have him on speakerphone.

The surgeon was holding a paper for her to sign off on the procedure, and he handed it to her.

"So, I've been looking at your imaging. Today I'm going to operate on your left leg, and I will rotate your femur fifteen degrees. Do you have any questions?" His words were fine, but as he explained the procedure, he did a hand motion indicating that he would be rotating her leg inward, not outward. As he continued, she looked at the form and noticed that the procedure reinforced his hand movement. It was written in for the wrong direction.

Brooke went pale. Finally, she spoke up.

"When we met in your office, my understanding is that you would be rotating my femur fifteen degrees to the *outside*, not the inside."

The surgeon stared at the young woman for a moment before looking again at his folder.

"Give me a minute, please," he said before pulling up his computer. After a long pause as he reviewed her imaging, he spoke again.

"You are correct," he announced. "I want to assure you that I now have your details correct, and I will be rotating your left leg as we discussed in clinic." He scratched out and corrected the details on the form, and she signed it.

Her dad on the other line didn't understand what was going on, since he hadn't seen the hand motion. If Brooke hadn't been very savvy about the details of her surgery, her leg would have been rotated in the wrong direction. (Imagine this happening to someone less educated on the details of their surgery, or for a procedure was more high-risk.)

Later that night when she was recovering in her overnight room, the surgeon tiptoed in to check on her—as he was known for his compassionate bedside manner. "You're looking great," he said. "And I just want you to know I rotated your leg the correct direction. This morning I had you confused with another case I had today."

While medical mistakes are not uncommon, this particular surgeon was in his seventies. Due to his experience, time on job, and commensurate salary, he booked multiple back-to-back procedures on surgery days so he could demonstrate his productivity (RVU) and justify his high income.

The Healthcare Matrix Determines Where Doctors Spend Their Time

From my role as an administrator and a clinician, I know firsthand how the amount of time doctors spend completing RVUs and other documentation has become increasingly onerous. Each day I must document things that have nothing to do with why I'm caring for a patient. When I get a letter from another doctor or a visit note about a patient's past medical history, I often must read ten-plus pages of documentation, all required by the insurance company to prove that each service I provide for a patient justifies the insurance payment.

While both serve critical roles, insurance and electronic medical records (EMRs) force doctors to work longer, harder hours. If a doctor doesn't bill for comprehensive care visits in great detail, they may not get paid for services they've provided. While seeing fifty patients a day, doctors often must bounce from patient rooms to laptops as they try to track down all the information they need for documentation. Since it's not possible to complete all of the documentation during an eight-hour workday, doctors spend their "time off" completing their documentation (more on this shortly).

EMRs also aren't ubiquitous; hospitals and clinics use various systems. And many of them don't communicate with one another.

The insurance companies dictate what must be documented for doctors to get paid, and then the government comes up with Medicaid and Medicare reimbursement that closely mirrors what the insurance companies demand. The healthcare providers have no say in the process. Doctors end up doing paperwork, filling out endless forms, and justifying their paychecks while patient care—the role doctors spent the first thirty-plus years of their lives preparing for—can seem like the lowest priority in the healthcare matrix.

The Healthcare Matrix Dictates Which Patients Doctors Treat

Some hospitals demand that physicians treat every patient, so the hospital system can receive reimbursement from the government. Emergency department (ED) doctors like my father were encouraged to see each patient, regardless of medical necessity, so the system could make more money. Yet this practice created two huge problems. First, the lack of gatekeeping over which patients get seen in the ED leads to patient dissatisfaction over long wait times. No hospital wants to read an online review announcing to the cyber-masses that "I had to wait four hours before they even took me back." Second, this practice burns out good doctors, not only because of the sheer volume of patients, but also because this practice turns the ED into an after-hours clinic.

My father wrote an op-ed piece for *Emergency Department News* where he argued against this practice imposed by hospital administrators. He said that a patient "needs to be seen in the right place at the right time by the right person." Someone with an earache doesn't likely belong at the ED; three a.m. is probably not the right time to seek treatment, and an emergency room physician isn't the best resource for such routine matters. Yet EDs across the country see patients who need nothing more than prescription re-fills because they ran out and didn't reach out to the doctor during business hours. In his op-ed piece, I could feel my father's burnout in his words.

The Healthcare Matrix Determines Which Medication Doctors Can Prescribe

Earlier I shared about a friend whose insurance company refused to cover pregabalin, a commonly prescribed medication for nerve pain. The insurance company would cover a less expensive drug, but that one didn't work for my friend.

Lest you think this is an isolated example, let me assure you that my friend isn't alone in his experiences. A 2021 survey found that 32 percent of those surveyed had an insurance company deny coverage for a needed medication. Another 31 percent were told by their insurance company that they needed to try a covered medication (or several) first to see if it worked before insurance would cover the prescribed medication (Fulton 2022).

The decision-makers on the health insurance side of the matrix supersede the expertise of trained physicians when it comes to what medication is best for each patient. This interplay forces doctors to become subject-matter experts in working around insurance companies or using less effective alternatives to a medication or treatment not covered by insurance.

Doctors find themselves stuck between doing everything within their power to treat each patient to the best of their ability and the multiple hoops set up by the insurance companies to maximize corporate profits.

The Healthcare Matrix Punishes Good Doctors in Poor Communities

Many rules, regulations, and policies add extra stress to the already fragmented healthcare system. The government requires metrics to demonstrate quality for performance in healthcare.

I'll use diabetes as an example. The government wants to know *how many patients with diabetes who were seen in the hospital met with a diabetic education specialist.* Based on the numbers reported, a hospital might receive some reimbursement from state and federal funding, Medicaid/Medicare dollars, and so on.

Quality standards are critical in healthcare; however, some of the performance standards that doctors fail to meet exist outside of their direct control. Doctors can experience *learned helplessness,* a psychological phenomenon where individuals experience negative consequences for situations outside of their control. After repeatedly trying and failing to be successful, many people simply quit trying.

For example, we closely monitor patients on dialysis to make sure their phosphorus remains within a certain range. When a patient's kidneys fail, they cannot remove excess phosphorus, which throws off the balance in the blood between phosphorus and calcium. As a result, the body leaches calcium from bones, making that person's bones brittle.

I can prescribe phosphate binders, medications designed to keep phosphorus levels in check. But those medications cannot fully compensate for patients who eat a diet high in phosphorus including foods like dairy, beans, and nuts. How can I be faulted for what a patient chooses to eat? I can educate my patients on the foods that make the DO NOT EAT list, but it's up to the patient to comply. The same holds true when a dialysis patient has low hemoglobin levels because they continually skip dialysis. At best, I can schedule an appointment with a patient and write them the prescription they need to stay healthy. But I don't have the power to make them show up for their appointments, fill their prescriptions, or take their medication as directed.

When a doctor fails to meet quality standards for factors out of their control, they feel hurt, stressed, and frustrated. Some doctors try to increase patient compliance by spending more time with each patient and slowly reviewing the treatment plan with them. As a result, the doctor's day gets longer, and their stress increases. And if they don't improve their numbers, the hospital doesn't get paid for work they've already done, which makes hospital administrators unhappy. This of course falls on the doctor, creating even more stress.

The current system is most unfair to doctors serving low socioeconomic populations. Again, I'll use the dialysis unit as an example. Disadvantaged patients are more likely than others to live in "food deserts" with limited access to fresh food because it is expensive; sadly, though, "food deserts" have limitless access to fast, cheap, preprepared foods. Dialysis alone cannot compensate for patients with poor diets. In other words, these patients struggle to follow dietary restrictions due to no fault of their own.

To keep costs low, the government wants as many dialysis patients as possible on home dialysis. While home dialysis is a great option for some patients, this isn't the best solution for patients with a limited education, those who share an apartment with ten other people, those who suffer from dexterity issues or poor eyesight, or those without a care partner to assist in the treatment. Yet doctors working with patients from low socioeconomic groups or other limitations are held to the same standard for the number of patients on home dialysis as providers in wealthy areas working in private practice. Academic institutions take the poorest patients and those most likely to have the worst clinical outcomes. Private practices don't touch these patients because these individuals don't generate money.

Equate these standards to a lawyer who wouldn't get paid if they lose a case. Would any lawyer take hard cases? The healthcare matrix created this tension, and it's the doctors who pay the price by working longer hours under increasing stress.

Keep in mind that those mandating technology like EMRs and establishing regulations are far removed from the patients being served. As such, many of their decisions are based on *what brings in or saves the most money* instead of *what's best for each individual patient*. EMR technology rarely considers those providing the actual care. Once again, always conscious of what brings in the most billing or reimbursement dollars, leaders in the healthcare matrix don't always keep the health and welfare of patients in the forefront of their decisions. And for healthcare professionals with a passion for caring for patients, the money-making system adds to their stress and disillusionment.

How Do Doctors Survive These Challenges?

As I've discussed, doctors didn't train to be leaders or to run healthcare like a business, nor were they trained in how to navigate the healthcare labyrinth to get their patients the necessary care. Like when Harry Truman became the accidental President of the United States, many doctors enter their professions completely in the dark about what the job entails. They don't know what decisions have already been made for them by an administration, nor do they understand how insurance companies and government regulations often interfere with providing the best treatment for their patients.

Early in this chapter, I shared the two ways that experienced doctors can justify their salaries. One, they can enter administration, or two, they can see more patients. Similarly, doctors can endure the responsibility of their roles in one of two ways. First, they can check out emotionally by choosing to go through the motions—checking boxes and doing what they're told as a survival technique. However, those doctors who choose to be passive followers are more likely to succumb to *burnout* or *compassion fatigue* (see sidebar for a brief introduction on these topics, and more on physician burnout in the next chapter).

Burnout is "a psychological syndrome of emotional exhaustion, depersonalization, and reduced personal accomplishment," a condition that affects half of all doctors and residents (CMA 2023). This exhaustion eats away at the soul and makes it difficult to impossible to manage everyday stressors.

Closely linked to burnout is *compassion fatigue.* A healthcare worker suffering from compassion fatigue may experience the following:

- Feeling overwhelmed, hopeless, helpless, or powerless when hearing of others' suffering
- Feelings of anger, irritability, sadness, and anxiety
- Feeling detached from their surroundings or from their physical or emotional experience
- Feeling emotionally, psychologically, or physically exhausted, burnt out or numb
- Physical symptoms such as nausea, dizziness, headaches
- Reduced empathy
- Feeling hypersensitive or insensitive to stories of human suffering
- Limited tolerance for stress
- Self-isolation and withdrawal
- Relationship conflict
- Feeling less efficient or productive at work
- Reduced pleasure in activities they used to enjoy
- Difficulty sleeping and nightmares

- Difficulty concentrating, focusing, or making decisions
- Self-medicating and an increase in substance use (CAMH 2023)

I've known doctors who survived by checking out emotionally and going through the motions, but this is a choice of default. Checking out comes with some heavy consequences. How can a physician stay fully engaged in a role where they watch people suffer but lack the ability to positively impact patients' health—alleviating their pain or treating their conditions? Not long. Doctors didn't power through years of medical training so they could feel powerless in positively shaping the lives of their patients.

I shared that doctors have two options to survive the challenges they face in practicing medicine. Checking out emotionally is one option, but it's not the only or best one. The other option is for doctors to strike the critical balance between patient care and bureaucratic duties.

Bryan Vartabedian, MD, serves as the Chief Pediatric Officer at Texas Children's Hospital North Austin. He recently wrote: "Three A's of physician success are availability, affability, and ability. In this order" (Vartabedian 2018). I agree with Dr. Vartabedian's assessment, with one caveat: add another A, administration.

Availability

"Showing up is half the battle" is a quote attributed to people ranging from Woody Allen to Stephen Hawking. Regardless of who may have said these words, the idea of being available when your patients have a medical need is critical for physicians. Obviously, emergency department doctors like my father have no idea what health issue the next patient coming through the hospital doors may need diagnosed and treated. But even specialty doctors who have reviewed a patient's charts don't always know what to expect in the office. In either case, a doctor must show up, take their time with patients, and be available to answer questions. A brilliant, world-class doctor with limited availability does less good for their patients than an average doctor who's available.

Affability

When someone says that their doctor has a "great bedside manner," they're saying their physician is affable. The fictitious character played by Hugh Laurie in the television series *House* was a perfect example of a doctor with intelligence but no human kindness. While Dr. House made for great comedic drama, few in the real world would tolerate his coldness.

Ability

Ability comes last for a reason. We've all heard the joke: *What do you call a doctor who finished last in their medical school class? Doctor.* Doctors engage in hundreds of hours of intensive classroom lectures, practicums, and on-the-job training. Yes, skill and experience levels vary from doctor to doctor. But a physician with less experience who shows up for patients with compassion will create positive patient perceptions and outcomes.

Administration

This is the fourth A that I think must be added to the list is administration. Why is it critical that doctors master the administrative part of the job? Doctors spend an average of 15.6 hours each week on paperwork and other administrative tasks, which amounts to more than three hours each day (Franklin 2021)! A time in motion study of doctors reported that physicians spend 27 percent of their time seeing patients and 49.2 percent of their time on administrative duties. That same study found that even while seeing patients in their office, they spend 37 percent of their time taking notes about the visit (Lee 2016)!

What kind of administrative duties? Correspondence with colleagues about patients, ensuring information is entered correctly into the patient's EMRs, coding visitation notes so that insurance companies cover the visit and/or medication, documentation for government reimbursement, and so on....

Unfortunately, doctors today can't fulfill their oath/declaration and provide the best care for their patients unless they master the administrative part of the job. Years ago, a doctor would write a prescription, rip it from their prescription pad, and hand it to the patient. Today, writing a prescription involves many steps, some to safeguard the patient and others to comply with insurance companies' requirements. Then the quality of care a doctor provides is measured on patient adherence to their treatment plan.

Is this work sexy? No. Is doing "paperwork" gratifying? No. Did doctors-in-training visualize spending nearly half of their days doing administrative work? Probably not. But unless a doctor embraces this necessary part of the role, their patients won't get the treatment they deserve.

I need to make one last point on the impact of the administrative work placed on doctors. Older doctors like my father practiced medicine before the advent of personal computers. The myriad of technological advancements and changes each year means these doctors have a steeper learning curve when it comes to using technology. They finished their formal education without playing video games, reading spreadsheets, having passwords required for every part of their lives, learning coding or programming, or even using the internet for research. Younger doctors have a clear advantage when it comes to embracing and mastering the technology used for much of the administrative part of the job. The effect this had on the older generation of doctors like my father has been greatly underappreciated.

How to Thrive Under Constant Pressure

Doctors have enough pressure trying to live up to the impossibly high standard of their oath/declaration. I therefore believe that doctors should "outsource" to experts as many non-medical parts of the job as possible instead of trying to become a master of all. Let's explore what can be outsourced to others.

Personal Finances

Not everyone has the time, aptitude, or desire to become the next Warren Buffett. That's OK. But that doesn't mean you are unable to take responsibility for your finances. Here are some ways to do that:

- Take a personal finance class in undergraduate school or online.
- Ask if your medical school offers a personal finance class (in my opinion, personal finance should be a prerequisite to starting medical school).
- Find a professional money manager (certified financial planner and/or financial advisor) to manage your finances for you.
- Hire a certified personal accountant (CPA) to help you with your taxes, at least at the start of your career so you can establish a norm for your filings.

Legal Assistance

Doctors are often stereotyped for their poor handwriting; lawyers are often stereotyped for writing contracts that no one understands. And you know the adage about lawyers, right? "A lawyer who represents himself has a fool for a client." Unless you went to law school (and as the adage suggests, *even if you went to law school),* don't try to serve as your own legal counsel.

When it comes to signing a work contract—

- Know the expectations for your productivity prior to signing, and
- Meet with a contract lawyer to ensure you understand everything you're committing to.

Mentorship

Beyond knowing what medical specialty you wish to pursue, you also must know what kind of doctor you wish to become. Those aren't the same things. The first involves your residency, fellowship, and additional formal training; the latter is about what traits you wish to exude in your work.

Find someone who makes the work look easy. Maybe that person has a calm, confident demeanor. Perhaps they seem to make better decisions than others. It could be that they always look rested and focused, or they have the kind of work-life balance you want in your own life. Once you decide the traits you wish to acquire and project, look for someone who has them. Then ask that person to mentor you.

An ideal mentor is one who can teach you things that aren't in textbooks or policy manuals. They can teach you informally; you can learn simply by asking questions and following their examples.

Resources

Medicine requires a cohesive team to provide the best care to patients. Doctors who try to go it alone often end up burnt out as well as disappointed with their results. The best doctors know how to identify, attract, and retain top employees. Additionally, they know the strengths and skills of those around them. This allows doctors to accumulate a pool of subject-matter experts to answer questions and help them.

Chapter 6 Summary

Great doctors who studied medicine to improve the quality of patient's lives can get disillusioned when the Hippocratic Oath bumps up against the reality of the healthcare matrix. Most doctors learn how to survive and even thrive once they understand how the game is played. But some of them languish along the way.

Many practicing physicians were top tier students from grade school through college. But good grades don't guarantee a happy-ever-after existence for physicians. In addition to intelligence, doctors need to admit when they would be better served by tapping into outside experts.

- Understand the basics of personal finance. Take classes, read books, or find a financial planner or advisor to guide you.
- Don't try to be your own lawyer. Fluency in medicalese doesn't translate into legalese. Find a lawyer to counsel you before you sign a work contract.
- Look for a physician that practices work-life balance and seems happy. Ask that person to mentor you in the art of living as a doctor.
- Build your "executive rolodex." Look for expert resources across various disciplines so you have handy experts for both medical and non-medical questions that you encounter.

In the next chapter, I'll explain the perfect storm that traps some doctors during their careers.

Doctors Don't Need to Succumb to the Perfect Storm

In late October of 1991, an area of low pressure developed off the coast of Atlantic Canada before turning into a strong cyclone. High winds slammed against the East Coast of the United States, generating strong waves that battered the coast. As the storm moved over warmer water, meteorologists classified it as a tropical storm. By November 1, the tropical storm morphed into a hurricane with sustained winds of over 75 miles per hour.

Two years later, author Sebastian Junger started writing a book about the storm. As part of his research, he worked with Bob Case of the National Weather Service to better understand the nature of the 1991 nor'easter. He learned that the storm coalesced around three different weather-related events (Chartuk 2000):

- A low-pressure system full of warm air
- A high-pressure system full of cool, dry air
- Hurricane Grace full of tropical moisture

When these three weather systems met, they formed what became known as *The Perfect Storm,* which serves as the title of Junger's best-selling 1997 book and the movie of the same name a few years later. The 1991 Halloween Storm, as it came to be called, sank the *Andrea Gail* and claimed the lives of its six crew members along with seven others on shore.

A similar perfect storm encircles many healthcare workers today. Healthcare professionals with underlying trauma, insufficient training in nonmedical areas of expertise, long hours, and endless demands of their job can find themselves in the path of a potential perfect storm.

I've already shared some of the stressors that many medical professionals struggle with:

- Unresolved childhood traumas
- The rigor of medical school and residency
- Entering the "real world" of medicine after residency
- Having a crisis of identity
- The inability to turn off work to lead a balanced life
- The ongoing increase in non-patient-facing administrative work

We all know people who have survived severe trauma, identity crises, and enormous work stress. We also know people who have overcome educational and experiential deficits to learn whatever they needed to be successful. However, the perfect storm brews when someone faces several of these issues at once. Unless a person is willing and able to manage their stress levels in these situations, they are prone to suffer from mental health issues as well as addiction.

Many doctors respond to stress like the prototypical strong, silent type, slipping on a façade like the old, classic stoic characters played by John Wayne, Gary Cooper, and Clint Eastwood. This is what my father did. Instead of showing vulnerability, expressing his emotions, or asking for help, my father suffered in silence—like countless other healthcare professionals do each day. A recent article states of physician suicide, "It's an alarming trend that is happening increasingly more often to our nation's healers….Pre-pandemic, there were reports of 300 to 400 physicians annually reported to have taken their lives. Anecdotally, the numbers were likely far higher then, and they are feared to be even higher now" (Feist 2021).

Suffering in silence can be deadly…like it was for my father.

After thoroughly researching the mental health pressures that doctors face, reporter Julia Belluz wrote, "Medicine is, ironically, a profession that punishes some doctors for getting mental health care. Many physicians work under intense pressure and are exposed to trauma on the job. A worrying number of doctors die by suicide each year. Yet structural barriers—enforced in part by medical boards and hospital systems—frequently discourage doctors from accessing care that could save their lives" (Belluz 2021). This lack of transparency is also thought to contribute to the underreporting of these physicians' cause of death.

I believe another issue leading to this underreporting of physician suicide is the stigma around admitting to mental health struggles, which I will discuss later in this chapter.

My Father Didn't Have to Die

Just writing, "My father didn't have to die," breaks my heart. My father didn't know how to overturn the traumas of his past, reverse the bad habits he had developed, and address his deteriorating mental health. Had he addressed each of these stressors that he faced—the ones I've listed in this book, along with their potential solutions—I wholeheartedly believe he would still be alive today.

My father's personal history put him at risk of developing addiction. According to research from the National Institute on Alcohol Abuse and Alcoholism, "Early-childhood trauma is strongly associated with developing mental health problems, including alcohol dependence, later in life" (Brady and Back 2012). As my father got older, he drank when he felt stressed. And then he drank when he wanted to *switch off* but lacked the skills to do it on his own.

My father wasn't unique in struggling with addiction. The National Library of Medicine estimates that 10 to 15 percent of all healthcare professionals will misuse drugs or alcohol at some time during their career. This number mirrors the general population; however, what makes this so troubling is that doctors are responsible for the health and well-being of their patients. Doctors commit enough human errors even without the addition of alcohol- or drug-impaired decisions that can negatively affect patient outcomes.

The most frequently abused drugs by healthcare professionals are benzodiazepines and opiates, with specialties such as anesthesia and emergency medicine carrying the highest rate of abuse. These medical specialists have a great amount of stress given the life-and-death nature of their work, and it's also possible that the rate of abuse coincides with the relative ease of access doctors have to these drugs (Baldisseri 2007).

Even in my father's time, some doctors developed problems with addiction while working as residents. How do you remain fully focused and alert despite working forty-eight- or seventy-two-hour days? Unfortunately, a subset of residents take stimulants to help them perk up and alcohol to bring them back down when they get the chance to sleep. Of course, not every resident or attending uses stimulants or alcohol to get through grueling times, but my dad eventually leaned on alcohol to "stabilize" his moods.

Coinciding with his addictions, my father suffered from mental health issues, which are increasingly common for doctors. In fact, *practicing physicians are more prone to suffer from mental health struggles than the general population.* A recent study found that 29 percent of physicians suffer from depression, double the rate of the non-doctor population in the US. Another study found that anxiety and depression for residents has reached nearly 50 percent (Hata 2022). Some of the increase in reported mental health challenges is due to the COVID-19 pandemic, but even prior to the pandemic, healthcare professionals struggled.

What contributes to the likelihood that a doctor will implode? Once again, family history, trauma, untreated anxiety or depression, low frustration tolerance, and an inability to manage stress can predispose a person to fall into a bottle of liquor or pills. While doctors face the same challenges as non-doctors—family, divorce, bills, children, and so on—they carry the additional stress of serving patients from within a fractured healthcare system.

Pain specialist and anesthesiologist Michael Sprintz described how the pressure of training and serving as a physician highlights any existing internal struggles a doctor might carry: "Medicine makes you more of who you already are."

Sprintz's expertise comes from more than practicing medicine. He entered medical school with unresolved childhood emotional trauma. He chose to study anesthesiology for several reasons: He had a deep knowledge of pharmacology and physiology, loved interventional procedures and the technology in the operating rooms, and quite simply, the practice of anesthesiology came naturally to him. Sprintz also had a genetic lineage primed for addiction, so Anesthesiology was a natural, unconsciously perfect fit. He started abusing substances when he was 13 and his addiction eventually included alcohol, propofol (known as "milk of amnesia"), amphetamine, fentanyl, ecstasy, marijuana and other drugs to help cope with his psychological pain. Fortunately, Sprintz entered recovery, dealt with addictive disease and his past traumas, and reentered the medical field to become a leading expert on the intersection of addiction and chronic pain (Carbonara and Sprintz 2023)."

But many doctors don't get help. One study found that 41 percent of doctors with mental health struggles reported that they refused to self-report their illnesses (Gerada 2018). Unlike people in other professions, physicians quickly learn to hide their problems. Many doctors fear that disclosing an addiction or mental health struggle may be career-ending.

The Perfect Storm Can Lead to the Misnomer Called "Burnout"

Mona Masood, MD, a psychiatrist specializing in working with healthcare professionals, believes she's found the reason that medicine attracts individuals more prone to suffer from mental health problems. She reports that *medicine attracts perfectionists,* those who put enormous pressure on themselves to succeed (Belluz 2021).

Washington University psychiatrist, Jessi Gold, MD, says, "Emotions, struggling, are an imperfection, and medicine is a field of perfection" (Masson).

Doctors believe they must be perfect. If they aren't perfect, a patient could die. If a student enters medical school without perfectionism in their DNA, they will quickly acquire this mindset by the time they enter residency. Talk about putting yourself under constant pressure! Unfortunately, this obsession with perfection can lead to what is commonly called *burnout*—a concept I introduced in the last chapter.

Burnout—as defined in the last chapter—describes the emotional, physical, and mental state someone enters when the pressure to perform is greater than the physical and emotional reserve to perform. Burnout is caused by excessive, prolonged stress—such as the pressure to be perfect every moment of the day or, as throughout the COVID pandemic, needing to work extended hours while short-staffed and fearful that they may bring the virus home to expose loved ones. Burnout symptoms include the following:

- Exhaustion
- Cynicism
- Decreased productivity
- A deep sense of failure
- Self-doubt
- Helplessness
- Detachment from others

Today, more than half of physicians report at least one of these symptoms (Talbot and Dean 2018).

Since doctors often believe they must be perfect, many resist the idea that they could succumb to burnout. As one author put it, burnout "suggests a failure of resourcefulness and resilience," negative attributes that physicians have spent years of rigorous training in a demanding role to combat. For these doctors, the idea of burnout means they aren't strong enough to be competent and immune to pressure.

But is a doctor's so-called lack of resourcefulness, resilience, and strength under relentless pressure really *burnout?* Or is the label of burnout actually "victim shaming." Instead of calling the condition that many doctors suffer from *burnout*, researchers Wendy Dean, MD, and Simon Talbot, MD, call it "moral injury." Dr. Zubin Damania says this about moral injury:

People go to war. They have a set of moral values. They care about other human beings. And then they are forced to either become a part of or bear witness to things that are so against everything they believe, that when they come back, they fall apart. We call it PTSD. We have a million names for it. What it is, is moral injury.

Humans are moral, idealistic creatures that resonate love for other humans. And what happens when our moral ideals meet the real world?....What happens when [they're] trained to give the best possible care regardless of socioeconomic status, race, condition, gender? But then [they] meet the real world where it's all about the insurance company's bottom line? It's all about the hospital system's revenue. It's all about throughputs and RVUs. And then [they] meet the electronic health record that is a glorified cash register with a little patient stuff tacked on.

How do you treat moral injury? You change the system (Damania 2019).

Psychiatrist Mona Masood summarizes the problem as this: "Our moral compass is incredibly compromised by the systemic barriers in the US that have made it about the bottom line rather than what we can do for patients" (Belluz 2021).

Moral Injury Can Be Fatal

In addition to suffering from untreated and undiagnosed mental health problems and dependance on alcohol for several years, my dad suffered from moral injury, a condition that I believe helps explain why doctors have the highest suicide across all professions (Wallace 2023). My father felt tormented by Adverse Childhood Experiences (ACEs), deteriorating mental health, financial setbacks, and growing addiction problems. And he grieved over his inability to provide the best care to his patients due to burdens placed upon him by the hospital system, creating moral injury that grew increasingly worse the longer he practiced medicine.

During his nearly thirty years working as an emergency department physician, Dr. Scott Jolley provided compassion and expertise to thousands of patients. But the pace and pressure of the job took its toll on his mental health. In 2018, the compassionate doctor referred to as "The Patriarch" for his wise, calm manner began locking horns with his colleagues. In 2018, his coworkers organized a meeting to discuss Jolley's anger issues. In his fifties, Jolley decided the time had come to step away from medicine, and he met with his administration about winding down his hours as he planned his retirement.

Enter COVID. Instead of his role shrinking, Jolley was assigned longer hours in the ER, often the nightshift. Due to cutbacks, Jolley worked alone. He requested additional doctor support on the busy night shift, but the hospital administration denied his request, along with his request to work pre-retirement hours since he had not yet reached the age of sixty.

Jolley took an unpaid sabbatical to try to restore his mental health. But this step increased his stress. Like my father, Jolley worried that he would lose his license and credentials. Additionally, he feared that his administration would learn if he saw a therapist and got a diagnosis for his struggles. He worried that he would be putting his career in jeopardy.

But eventually he sought help. He was diagnosed with PTSD and placed on medication to treat his depression and anxiety. During this time, Jolley attempted suicide. He was admitted to the psychiatric unit of his own hospital. His insurance company would only cover treatment provided within the hospital system. In the psychiatric unit, Jolley was treated by his friends and colleagues. Not only was Jolley's condition now common knowledge among his peers, but his hospital room had no doors.

Jolley was discharged two days later to return home feeling broken, exposed, and full of shame. Two weeks later, he took his own life.

Jolley's wife believes that the medical profession failed her husband who wanted nothing more than to save lives. Before Jolley died by suicide, he had asked, in writing, for his hospital's administration for help five times. Known for his compassion, and with no previous history of mental illness, Dr. Scott Jolley died from moral injury and a broken system.

"They had a business to run and wanted to survive the pandemic and didn't recognize Scott was reaching out for help," his wife said. "He told me they all thought he was just an old, angry doctor" (Belluz 2021).

Looking back, I see signs that my dad had problems. But he worked hard to cover his emotional state and the damage he felt inside.

I didn't learn about this situation when it happened, but people at work started to realize that alcohol was becoming a problem for my dad. My father knew that if the hospital reported him to the medical board, he could lose his medical license. Not knowing if the hospital would report him, Dad "self-reported" that he had a problem. By self-reporting, he hoped to avoid the worst consequences. The hospital spent several days arranging to cover my dad's shifts...until they met with him, suspended him, and investigated the allegation.

At the time, Dad was one of the few people in his geographic area with his expertise. The hospital needed him, and my father committed to doing whatever he must do to get beyond the allegation and recover his reputation. Since he self-reported, my father was required to go to treatment and attend counseling. Within three or four months, he went back to practicing medicine.

But nothing else changed.

Workers in these professions are more likely to be at risk for depression and suicide:

- Doctors
- Nurses
- Emergency medical technicians (EMTs)
- Veterinarians
- Humanitarian workers
- Lawyers
- Construction workers
- Childcare workers
- Restaurant workers

Many of the professions listed come with higher-than-average student loan debt, long hours, staff shortages, and/or close proximity to human (or animal) suffering. Others suffer from low wages and job insecurity (Akhtar and Aydin 2019).

Then his outward troubles started again, and he was immediately placed on administrative leave. He later wrote in one of his good-bye notes, "You know I could have never endured the shame and embarrassment of a suspension."

My dad considered the three likely outcomes of his second offense. One, they could report him to the board, putting his license at risk. Two, they could send him back to counseling. Or three, they could fire him.

My dad never wanted anyone in the family, other than my mother, to learn what had happened at work. Instead, he carried the heavy weight of his shame alone.

If you're having difficulty understanding how my father felt as he faced a second offense for drinking and the potential end of his career, let me describe what it feels like when a doctor falls from grace. As I've already explained, doctors are trained to be perfect. Anything short of perfection could put a life at risk. In addition to risking the life of a patient, imperfection can lead to lawsuits, a constant threat that doctors live under with each patient they see. If a doctor overlooks something during the patient exam, fails to ask the right questions, misses a symptom, inaccurately diagnoses a problem, or prescribes the wrong medication, that doctor has a target on their back for a lawsuit.

Emergency department doctors like my father work under a heightened fear of lawsuits. People go to the ED for emergencies, so every patient is potentially at high risk. My father loved the adrenaline of not knowing what medical problem might show up in the next patient who walked through the doors of the hospital. *Will it be an ear infection? An aneurysm? A heart attack?* But as much as he loved the fast pace of the ED and the life-and-death decisions he made each day, he feared getting sued. His stress came from not only wanting to do the best thing for each patient, but also from the potential consequences on his livelihood should he make an error.

I believe that once my father got placed on administrative leave the second time, he walked out of the hospital knowing what he would do. In *Why People Die by Suicide,* Dr. Thomas Joiner outlines three conditions that must be met for a person to be considered high risk for attempting and dying by suicide:

1. They must feel they are a burden to others.
2. They must feel that they no longer belong.
3. They must acquire the ability to carry out a lethal plan (termed *learned fearlessness*).

My father met all three conditions. He didn't wish to disappoint or burden his family with his behavior or its consequences. Additionally, he felt that he was no longer fit for his job...or for life. Finally, as an ED doctor who had treated the aftermath of attempted or competed deaths by suicide, and who was a gun collector, he knew enough to make sure that he had the means to be successful with ending his own life.

My dad wrote long letters to each family member.

"This is the saddest day of my life. Not the day I die but the day before I die. I have to write these terrible letters. I could not begin to list all the things I did wrong in our marriage," his note to my mother began. *"Even though you might forgive me for all of it, I cannot forgive myself."*

To me he wrote, "Kathy, my first child, I was so proud. I am still proud of all you have accomplished and for the person you are...."

He explained his state of mind.

I have been suffering a major depression with possible "psychotic" features. I have mood swings and irrational behavior for no apparent reason. None of it seems to be goal-directed....I don't mean to blame all of the bad things in my life on mental illness, but I know that something is wrong. The ADD meds help, but I still find myself unable to focus or complete tasks at times. I get confused about all the patients.

The situation with me had to end sooner or later. If it wasn't this episode, it would eventually be something else. I live on the edge with risky behaviors, and I can't even see it. All of this will pass, and in two or three years you won't even mention my name. I will fade in your memory just like you mother, father, and my mother and father. They have ceased to exist as we know them.

He got his finances in order. He had already planned his funeral. He spent the next three days planning out how he would end his life.

Feeling enormous guilt and shame, my father never wished to look into the eyes of his loved ones and see an expression that told him that he was a failure, so he left nothing to chance. A blood alcohol level of .08 percent is considered legally impaired, and anyone found driving with this much alcohol in their system will be arrested. My father's blood alcohol level at the time of his death was .586 percent, more than seven times the legal limit. Blood alcohol levels above .40 percent often prove fatal. He also had taken large doses of amphetamines (Adderall), phenylpropanolamine (cold medicine similar to ephedrine), Cyclobenzaprine (muscle relaxer), and Benadryl. Just to ensure he would be successful this time, he then used a firearm to end his life. Missing from his toxicology report was his prescription antidepressant in therapeutic concentrations (i.e., he was not taking them).

"I didn't think he'd go through with it," one of my friends told me after my dad's death.

"What do you mean?" I asked.

"I mean, after the last time he tried to kill himself, I never imagined he'd try it again."

"What do you mean *after the last time*?" I asked, shocked and deeply troubled.

And that was how I learned that five years earlier, my father had gotten drunk, called 911, and then tried to shoot himself. But he was too drunk to pull the trigger. By the time EMS arrived, he had already passed out but still held the gun in his hand. The EMS personnel never took him to the hospital; my father was the medical director of EMS. And the incident was never reported.

Like my father, Sprintz didn't put up his hand to ask for help. Instead, his drug use got uncovered while finishing his second year of anesthesiology residency at Johns Hopkins. Once he was caught, his bosses sent him to a treatment program to get help. Initially, Sprintz went along with the program with one thought in his mind: *get back to medicine*. He didn't conquer his addictions overnight. But with work, he eventually reached a breakthrough in his recovery, and now with over 23 years in recovery, he's spent the last decade helping others overcome addictions and create better lives for themselves.

But unlike my father, Sprintz didn't suffer from underlying depression.

"Were you ever suicidal?" he was asked in an interview.

"Never," he answered emphatically. "I think I loved myself too much to ever take my own life. But when I was still in my addiction, I used [drugs], knowing that I might die. And I accepted that risk. My perspective was, 'if it happens, oh well.' But I didn't *want* to die."

"Did you ever suffer from depression?" he was asked.

"No. And thank God I didn't. If I'd had underlying depression, I'm sure that I would have considered suicide as an option, especially once my addiction blew up the career I'd spent years to build" (Carbonara and Sprintz 2023).

We're all familiar with the saying "the straw that broke the camel's back." As a beast of burden, camels possess incredible strength. They can carry 900 pounds on their backs while traveling twenty-five miles each day. They can also run as fast as a racehorse (SPANA 2023). But regardless of their power and speed, camels have their limits. The oft-repeated saying means that a person carrying even a light burden—over time and given the additional burdens they may be carrying already—can experience significant damage. My father had the burden of depression and what he described as a "psychotic" break. He added alcohol to his problem, distorting his thinking further. Prior to his being reported at work, he had lost his 401k, a situation that my father wrote about in the farewell letter to my mom, describing that moment as when he "lost hope." Each straw contributed to his decision to take his own life.

Avoiding the Perfect Storm

I've left many things to unpack from this chapter. Let me start by stating the obvious: not everyone suffering from unresolved childhood trauma, addiction, mental health issues, and moral injury will end up like my father. Additionally, not every medical school student and resident will suffer from long-term stress from their experiences.

However, some doctors will get hit by the perfect storm. Since it's impossible to determine which doctors will unravel under the demands of the job, my suggestions are broad and meant to help all doctors maintain strong mental health. (Most of this book has included solutions that you as a physician can implement. Now I'm going to include some that may involve changes to your organization's policies and procedures.)

Mandatory Annual Mental Health Screening

The Federal Aviation Administration (FAA) requires that pilots undergo a physical and mental health screening every six months to five years, depending on the pilot's age and type of flying they do. Given the potential consequences if a mentally ill pilot were to fly a passenger plane, these screenings make good sense to safeguard travelers.

Sadly, no agency requires doctors to pass a similar screening.

Some seasoned medical doctors would balk at such a requirement and deem it unnecessary. However, I think this needs to change immediately. Providing the best care to patients requires that their caregivers are mentally strong and well. All US hospital systems and most private practices offer Employee Assistance Programs (EAPs) where struggling employees can meet with an outside professional about mental health challenges. However, having EAP available is different than making it mandatory. Trained professionals can not only provide guidance and support, but they can also identify stressors and struggles that a client may underreport.

Provide Regular In-Service Training on Mental Health and Self-Care

Even though doctors complete a rotation in psychiatric care as part of residency, the short amount of time they spend doing rounds is insufficient to help doctors diagnose and treat themselves. Besides, every doctor knows that doctors make terrible patients. They think they know better than the doctor examining them!

Instead of cramming more training into the already-packed medical school and residency curriculum, hospital administrators must bring in-house training to their doctors. While this idea makes sense to laypeople and healthcare professionals alike, hospital administrators must be willing to make mental health and self-care learning a priority, even though taking doctors off rounds will impact their RVUs and patient volumes.

Hospital systems must take the lead in offering training on-site for their healthcare workers. The American Medical Association (AMA) needs to prioritize mental health training for the doctors they serve. The purpose of the AMA is to promote the science and art of medicine and the betterment of public health. But doctors can't give what they don't possess. By educating their membership on how to care for their personal and collective mental health, the AMA can best shape the betterment of public health. Mentally healthy doctors can compassionately identify and intervene on behalf of the patients they serve.

The best training for doctors includes case studies, research findings, and stories. Additionally, training should provide tips for how to talk with a colleague that you might be concerned about.

Remove the Stigma for Getting Help for Mental Illness and Substance Use Disorders

While treatments and medications have changed significantly over the last several decades, one part of medicine has gone unchanged: a doctor seeking help for a mental health or substance misuse problem might see their career disappear.

Licensure requirements vary by state, but most require doctors to fill out a questionnaire that includes questions about their mental health before obtaining a license. For example, a doctor must complete a licensure questionnaire in Alaska that asks twenty-five questions about their mental health, including, "Have you ever been diagnosed with, treated for, or do you currently have" followed by a list of mental health conditions ranging from depression, seasonal affective disorder, and "any condition requiring chronic medical or behavioral treatment" (Townsley and Katta 2023).

Imagine you're in your thirties. You've invested years in advanced education and are now heavily in debt without money or retirement savings. Now you're asked to complete a questionnaire that could determine if you will or will not be able to practice medicine, something you've spent one-third of your life preparing to do. Are you going to be honest about your past or present mental health struggles?

A recent study estimates that three hundred to four hundred physicians die by suicide each year. Probably linked to a doctor's knowledge of how to end their lives, they have a much higher death-by-suicide completion-to-attempt ratio than any other profession (Matheson 2023).

How many of these doctors showed signs of depression or, like my father, psychotic episodes? How many of them could have been pulled back from the brink had they gotten help or if a trusted colleague or family member had intervened?

As long as the medical establishment threatens the livelihoods of good doctors when they ask for help, the physician mental health problem will continue. Suicides will continue.

All of us should lobby legislators at the state level to remove invasive questions about mental health on licensure requirements. Thirty-one states ask similar questions for licensure to Alaska. Removing stigmatizing language is a small change that can make a huge difference in the lives of doctors. A treated mental health condition should not be viewed in the same light as an untreated one. Punitive laws and regulations make it nearly impossible for doctors to self-report out of fear of losing their medical licenses. Alternatively, doctors should be provided with other non-stigmatized or career-threatening options for seeking help when they need it.

Seek Confidential Help

Earlier in this chapter I shared the story of Scott Jolley, who self-reported his struggles to his hospital administration. When he got no relief from his appeal, he attempted to take his own life, landing him in the psychiatric unit inside of the very hospital where he worked in the ED. Humiliated, exposed, and full of shame, he took his own life a couple of weeks after he was discharged from treatment. In my view, his employer and the insurance company failed him.

Prompted by the chaos that ensued at the beginning of the COVID-19 pandemic, Mona Masood created the Physician Support Line as "a national peer-to-peer service provided by volunteer psychiatrists who are unapologetically supporting their physician and medical student colleagues on the many intersections of their personal and professional lives." While COVID served as the catalyst for the Physician Support Line, this service is also invaluable to doctors struggling with any problem (Bernard 2023).

This support line saves lives. Its peer-to-peer support is available to medical students, resident/fellows, attending physicians, and retired physicians. The calls are confidential, and nothing shared with the volunteers gets reported anywhere. The hotline requires no appointment and is open Monday through Friday from 8 a.m. to midnight.

Masood explains that the trained, licensed psychiatrist volunteer who answers the phones will talk with callers "about anything from being burned out to our frustrations with the health care system, including moral injury of what we thought we were going to be as physicians and who we turned out to be, and how that feels like some moral reckoning. We talk about family, and we talk about marriages. We talk about loneliness, sleep, isolation, and anything under the sun. It doesn't have to be a crisis to call" (Bernard 2023).

Keep this phone number handy for yourself and pass it on to any colleague you believe to be struggling: *1-888-409-0141.*

Chapter 7 Summary

Even those with the best lives will experience some emotional struggles, temporary setbacks, and periods of sadness. Some will go on to face anxiety, depression, addiction, suicidal thoughts (including ideation and suicide attempts), or even death by suicide. Unique to doctors, soldiers, and other first responders is the likelihood of experiencing moral injury. Yet as I shared earlier in the chapter, doctors are more prone to take their own lives than those working in any other profession.

The perfect storm for doctors and healthcare workers isn't usually one simple event; rather, healthcare professionals may encounter wave after complex wave of events arising from the nature of their work. As a society, we need to elevate the mental health crisis that many physicians face by enacting common-sense solutions.

- Mandatory annual mental health screenings can provide early identification of and intervention with doctors who are undergoing significant stress.
- Hospital systems and membership groups like the AMA must prioritize building the mental health of their employees and members.
- Adding mental health training also helps remove the stigma associated with doctors seeking help with mental illness, substance use disorders, and suicidal ideation. Shame doesn't cure the struggles that doctors experience; instead, shame forces doctors to go underground with their struggles, which further exacerbates the problem.

We all must advocate for doctors to tap into professional, confidential help. Fear of punishment and job loss currently keeps doctors silent. And silence can turn deadly.

Conclusion: A Call to Action

The issue of physician suicide has been ignored for too long. I wrote this book not only to shed light on the issue and tell my father's story, but also in writing this book, I found a path to healing. When my father died by suicide, I wondered if I would succumb to the same fate. After all, I'm a physician too. I asked myself, *Is this genetic? Do I have—or will I have—a mental illness?*

Writing out my thoughts and feelings—while researching the topic of physician mental health and suicide—helped me understand my father's struggles and the medical system's complacency in his death far more than I ever did before. Fortunately, I now know that I will not go down his path, but others will unless we do something.

Consider *First Do No Harm: A Physicians Mental Health Survival Guide from Medical School to Retirement* a call to action.

Those in medical school or a residency program, or those practicing medicine, can practice the principles shared here and avoid the same outcome as my father. My hope is that you will thrive in your practice, and that these proactive tools and strategies will help you.

But the issue of physician mental health, addiction, and suicide is bigger than you or me. Healthcare administrators, other doctors, and other medical professionals must:

- Talk about physician mental health, addiction, and suicide to remove the stigma attached to them.

- Demand changes in the healthcare system to remove moral injury and allow doctors to care for all patients.
- Make self-care a priority for those entrusted with overseeing the health and well-being of patients.

Together we can combat the growing epidemic of physician mental health, addiction, and suicide.

I've given presentations at many national venues about my father's story and the lessons I've learned, and I plan to continue to do so. My wish is that others can learn from my father's mistakes so his death may have as much meaning as his life did. While my father couldn't treat or heal himself, I want his death to save the life of anyone else who is struggling today.

If I can prevent one physician death from telling his story, then it is worth every single tear I have shed while writing it.

Bibliography

Agarwal, Pragya. 2020. *Sway: Unravelling Unconscious Bias*. London, UK: Bloomsbury Sigma.

Akhtar, Allana, and Rebecca Aydin. 2019. "Some of the Jobs Most at Risk for Suicide and Depression Are the Most Important to Society. Here's a Rundown of Mental-Health Risks for Doctors, Childcare Workers, First Responders, and More." Business Insider. November 14, 2019. https://www.businessinsider.com/jobs-with-mental-health-risks-like-suicide-depression-2019-10.

Asch, David A., Justin Grischkan, and Sean Nicholson. 2020. "Lower the Cost of Producing Doctors, Not Just the Price of Going to Medical School." STATNews. STAT. July 21, 2020. https://www.statnews.com/2020/07/21/lower-cost-producing-doctors-not-just-price-medical-school/.

Aupperle, Robin L., Andrew J. Melrose, Murray B. Stein, and Martin P. Paulus. 2012. "Executive Function and PTSD: Disengaging from Trauma." *Neuropharmacology* 62 (2): 686–94. https://doi.org/10.1016/j.neuropharm.2011.02.008.

"Average Hours Employed People Spent Working on Days Worked by Day of Week." 2023. U.S. Bureau of Labor Statistics. US Department of Labor. 2023. https://www.bls.gov/charts/american-time-use/emp-by-ftpt-job-edu-h.htm.

Baldisseri, Marie R. 2007. "Impaired Healthcare Professional." *Critical Care Medicine* 35 (Suppl): 106–16. https://doi.org/10.1097/01.ccm.0000252918.87746.96.

Belluz, Julia. 2021. "The Doctors Are Not All Right." Vox. Vox Media. June 23, 2021. https://www.vox.com/22439911/doctors-mental-health-suicide-coronavirus-pandemic.

Bernard, Rebekah. 2023. "Healing the Healer: The Physician Support Line." Medical Economics. *Medical Economics Journal.* May 1, 2023. https://www.medicaleconomics.com/view/healing-the-healer-the-physician-support-line.

Brady, Kathleen, and Sudie E. Back. 2012. "Childhood Trauma, Posttraumatic Stress Disorder, and Alcohol Dependence." Alcohol Research: Current Reviews 34 (4): 408–13.

Brown, Andy. 2021. "What to Expect During Your First Year of Residency." The DO. American Osteopathic Association. March 17, 2021. https://thedo.osteopathic.org/2021/03/what-to-expect-during-your-first-year-of-residency/.

Buga, Stephanie. 2021. "What Residency Is like in the U.S." The Daily Checkup. AMOpportunities. February 11, 2021. https://blog.amopportunities.org/2021/02/11/heres-what-to-expect-during-u-s-medical-residency/.

"Burnout." 2023. CMA.Ca. Canadian Medical Association. 2023. https://www.cma.ca/physician-wellness-hub/topics/burnout.

Booren, Steve. 2023. *Blind Spots: The Mental Mistakes Investors Make.* Greenwood Village, CO: Prosperion Financial Advisors.

Carbonara, Scott, and Michael Sprintz. 2023. Interview with Michael Sprintz. Personal.

Carbonara, Scott and Randy Grimes. 2022. Interview with Randy Grimes. Personal.

Chartuk, Bob. 2000. "NOAA Meteorologist Bob Case, The Man Who Named The Perfect Storm." NOAA News Online. National Weather Service. June 16, 2000. https://web.archive.org/web/20110716220940/http:/www.noaanews.noaa.gov/stories/s444.htm.

Chaudron, Linda H. MD, Harris, Toi MD, Chatterjee, Archana MD, PhD, and Lautenberger, Diana M. "Power Reimagined: Advancing Women Into Emerging Leadership Positions." *Academic Medicine* 98 (6):p 661-663, June 2023.

Chiaravalloti, Deborah. 2019. "The Origins of Common Medical Terminology and Acronyms." BoardVitals Blog. BoardVitals. March 6, 2019. https://www.boardvitals.com/blog/origins-medical-terminology-acronyms/.

Christensen, Tricia. 2023. "What Percent of the US Population Do Doctors Comprise?" United States Now. April 24, 2023. https://www.unitedstates-now.org/what-percent-of-the-us-population-do-doctors-comprise.htm.
Cohen, Jared. 2020. *Accidental Presidents: Eight Men Who Changed America*. New York, NY: Simon & Schuster.

Damania, Zubin. 2019. "It's Not Burnout, It's Moral Injury." ZDoggMD. March 8, 2019. https://zdoggmd.com/moral-injury/.

"Discover 13 Fun Facts about Camels." 2023. SPANA. Society for the Protection of Animals Abroad. April 27, 2023. https://spana.org/blog/13-fun-facts-about-camels/.

"Estimate Future College Costs with the College Cost Projector." 2023. Massachusetts Educational Financing Authority. 2023. https://www.mefa.org/pay/college-cost-projector.

Feist, J. Corey. 2021. "Physicians Suffering in Silence." Morning Consult. July 14, 2021. https://morningconsult.com/opinions/physicians-suffering-in-silence/.

"Fighting for the Victims of Fatigue & Overwork on the Road." 2023. Arnold & Itkin LLP. 2023. https://www.arnolditkin.com/houston-truck-accident-lawyer/truck-driver-fatigue/.

Finnegan, Joanne. 2016. "Thousands of Newly Graduated Doctors Don't Find a Residency Program Match." Fierce Healthcare. May 31, 2016. https://www.fiercehealthcare.com/practices/thousands-newly-graduated-doctors-don-t-find-a-residency-program-match.

Fork, Heather. 2020. "Leaving Medicine—Danielle's Story." Doctor's Crossing. September 25, 2020. https://doctorscrossing.com/leaving-medicine-danielles-story/.

Franklin, Remy. 2021. "Are Doctors Spending Less Time with Patients?" Mobius MD. October 9, 2021. https://mobius.md/2021/10/09/how-much-time-do-physicians-spend-with-patients/.

Fulton, Alex. 2022. "Survey Says: Insurance Providers May Put up Barriers to Care." HealthyWomen. July 18, 2022. https://www.healthywomen.org/created-with-support/insurance-providers-may-put-up-barriers-to-care.

Gerada, Clare. "Doctors, Suicide and Mental Illness." BJPsych bulletin, August 2018. https://www.ncbi.nlm.nih.gov/pmc/articles/PMC6436060.

Goebert, Deborah, Diane Thompson, Junji Takeshita, Cheryl Beach, Philip Bryson, Kimberly Ephgrave, Alan Kent, Monique Kunkel, Joel Schechter, and Jodi Tate. 2009. "Depressive Symptoms in Medical Students and Residents: A Multischool Study." *Academic Medicine* 84 (2): 236–41. https://doi.org/10.1097/acm.0b013e31819391bb.

Gupta, Nishtha, Sana Dhamija, Jaideep Patil, and Bhushan Chaudhari. 2021. "Impact of COVID-19 Pandemic on Healthcare Workers." *Industrial Psychiatry Journal* 30 (3): 282–84. https://doi.org/10.4103/0972-6748.328830.

Han, Zoe. 2022. "Fewer than 50% of U.S. Adults Are Now Married. It's Time to Give More Legal and Financial Breaks to Single People, Law Professor Says." MarketWatch. October 5, 2022. https://www.marketwatch.com/story/fewer-than-50-of-u-s-adults-are-now-married-its-time-to-give-more-legal-and-financial-breaks-to-single-people-law-professor-says-11664992681.

Hanson, Melanie. 2023. "Average Student Loan Debt [2023]: By Year, Age & More." Education Data Initiative. May 22, 2023. https://educationdata.org/average-student-loan-debt.

Hata, Susan. 2022. "Many Doctors Suffer from Anxiety and Depression. States Aren't Helping." BostonGlobe.Com. The Boston Globe. January

27, 2022. https://www.bostonglobe.com/2022/01/27/opinion/many-doctors-suffer-anxiety-depression-states-arent-helping/.

"How Common Is PTSD in Children and Teens?" 2018. Va.Gov. US Department of Veterans Affairs. September 18, 2018. https://www.ptsd.va.gov/understand/common/common_children_teens.asp.

"How Many Years of Postgraduate Training Do Surgical Residents Undergo?" 2023. FACS. American College of Surgeons. 2023. https://www.facs.org/for-medical-professionals/education/online-guide-to-choosing-a-surgical-residency/guide-to-choosing-a-surgical-residency-for-medical-students/faqs/training/.

"The Importance of Social Relationships to Physical and Mental Health." 2021. High Country Behavioral Health. January 18, 2021. https://www.hcbh.org/blog/posts/2021/january/the-importance-of-social-relationships-to-physical-and-mental-health/.

"Is There a Cost to Protecting, Caring for and Saving Others? Beware of Compassion Fatigue." 2023. CAMH.Ca. Centre for Addiction and Mental Health. 2023. https://www.camh.ca/en/camh-news-and-stories/is-there-a-cost-to-protecting-caring-for-and-saving-others-beware-of-compassion-fatigue.

"I'm a Doctor, Not a…" n.d. Memory Alpha. Fandom.com. Accessed June 1, 2023. https://memory-alpha.fandom.com/wiki/I%27m_a_doctor,_not_a...

Kroll, Michele M. 2022. "Prolonged Social Isolation and Loneliness Are Equivalent to Smoking 15 Cigarettes a Day." UNH Extension. University of New Hampshire. May 2, 2022. https://extension.unh.edu/blog/2022/05/prolonged-social-isolation-loneliness-are-equivalent-smoking-15-cigarettes-day.

Lee, Bruce Y. 2016. "Doctors Wasting over Two-Thirds of Their Time Doing Paperwork." Forbes. Forbes Magazine. September 7, 2016. https://www.forbes.com/sites/brucelee/2016/09/07/doctors-wasting-over-two-thirds-of-their-time-doing-paperwork/?sh=48170a2f5d7b.

Malito, Alessandra. 2019. "Are You Tired of Marie Kondo's 'Does It Spark Joy' Question? Here Are 5 Other Ways to Declutter." MarketWatch. January 19,

2019. https://www.marketwatch.com/story/tired-of-marie-kondos-decluttering-philosophy-here-are-5-smart-ways-to-unload-your-junk-2019-01-15.

Masson, Gabrielle. 2021. "Imperfection in a Field of Perfection: Why Some Physicians Don't Get Mental Health Treatment." Beckers Hospital Review. June 24, 2021. https://www.beckershospitalreview.com/hospital-physician-relationships/imperfection-in-a-field-of-perfection-why-some-physicians-don-t-get-mental-health-treatment.html

Matheson, John. 2023. "Physician Suicide." ACEP.Org. American College of Emergency Physicians. 2023. https://www.acep.org/life-as-a-physician/wellness/wellness/wellness-week-articles/physician-suicide/.

Medical Economics Staff. 2016. "5 Myths About Doctors Our Society Believes." MedicalEconomics.Com. *Medical Economics Journal*. July 28, 2016. https://www.medicaleconomics.com/view/5-myths-about-doctors-our-society-believes.

Medical Economics Staff. 2019. "The Top 10 Challenges Facing Physicians in 2020." *Medical Economics Journal*, December 10, 2019.

Mian, Amir, Dahye Kim, Duane Chen, and Wendy L. Ward. 2018. "Medical Student and Resident Burnout: A Review of Causes, Effects, and Prevention." *Journal of Family Medicine and Disease Prevention* 4 (4). https://doi.org/10.23937/2469-5793/1510094.

Miller, G.E. 2023. "The US Is the Most Overworked Nation in the World." 20somethingfinance.Com. January 10, 2023. https://20somethingfinance.com/american-hours-worked-productivity-vacation/.

Mindful Staff. 2020. "What Is Mindfulness?" Mindful.Org. July 8, 2020. https://www.mindful.org/what-is-mindfulness/.

Mineo, Liz. 2017. "Over Nearly 80 Years, Harvard Study Has Been Showing How to Live a Healthy and Happy Life." Harvard Gazette. Harvard University. April 11, 2017. https://news.harvard.edu/gazette/story/2017/04/over-nearly-80-years-harvard-study-has-been-showing-how-to-live-a-healthy-and-happy-life/.

Moore, Rebecca. 2019. "Survey Says: If You Didn't Have to Work, Would You?" PLANSPONSOR. ISS Media. March 4, 2019. https://www.plansponsor.com/survey-says-didnt-work/.

Morgan, Kate. 2021. "Why We Define Ourselves by Our Jobs." BBC Worklife. BBC. April 13, 2021. https://www.bbc.com/worklife/article/20210409-why-we-define-ourselves-by-our-jobs.

Morin, Amy. 2022. "4 Types of Parenting Styles and Their Effects on Kids." Edited by Ann-Louise T. Lockhart. Verywell Family. Dotdash Meredith. August 9, 2022. https://www.verywellfamily.com/types-of-parenting-styles-1095045.

"Name It to Tame It: Label Your Emotions to Overcome Negative Thoughts." 2022. Mindfulness.Com. June 29, 2022. https://mindfulness.com/mindful-living/name-it-to-tame-it.

Nomad Health. 2018. "Complete List of Average Doctor Salaries by Specialty." Nomad Health. Medium. April 11, 2018. https://medium.com/nomad-health/complete-list-of-average-doctor-salaries-by-specialty-e2bbbc0a6186.

Peterson, Sarah. 2018. "Effects." The National Child Traumatic Stress Network. CMHS/SAMHSA. March 31, 2018. https://www.nctsn.org/what-is-child-trauma/trauma-types/complex-trauma/effects.

Ponio, Ashley Anne. 2023. "Medical School Dropout Rate." TheMDJourney. April 21, 2023. https://themdjourney.com/medical-school-dropout-rate/.

Primack, Brian A., Terri C. Dilmore, Galen E. Switzer, Cindy L. Bryce, Deborah L. Seltzer, Jie Li, Douglas P. Landsittel, Wishwa N. Kapoor, and Doris M. Rubio. 2010. "Brief Report: Burnout Among Early Career Clinical Investigators." *Clinical and Translational Science* 3 (4): 186–88. https://doi.org/10.1111/j.1752-8062.2010.00202.x.

Probasco, Jim. 2023. "25 Highest Paid Occupations in the US." Investopedia. Dotdash Meredith. March 30, 2023. https://www.investopedia.com/personal-finance/top-highest-paying-jobs/.

Riffkin, Rebecca. 2014. "In US, 55% of Workers Get Sense of Identity from Their Job." Gallup.Com. Gallup. August 22, 2014. https://news.gallup.com/poll/175400/workers-sense-identity-job.aspx.

Roncero, Alexia. 2021. "How to Heal from Childhood Trauma: 3 Steps to Start Coping." BetterUp. December 29, 2021. https://www.betterup.com/blog/childhood-trauma.

Rymanowicz, Kylie. 2018. "Adverse Childhood Experiences (Aces): What Are They and How Can They Be Prevented?" Child & Family Development. Michigan State University Extension. December 13, 2018. https://www.canr.msu.edu/news/adverse-childhood-experiences.

Sanfey, Hilary, John A. Fromson, John Mellinger, Jan Rakinic, Michael Williams, and Betsy Williams. 2015. "Residents in Distress: An Exploration of Assistance-Seeking and Reporting Behaviors." *The American Journal of Surgery* 210 (4): 678–84. https://doi.org/10.1016/j.amjsurg.2015.05.011.

Schulz, Marc, and Robert Waldinger. 2023. "An 85-Year Harvard Study on Happiness Found the No. 1 Retirement Challenge That 'No One Talks About.'" CNBC. NBC. March 10, 2023. https://www.cnbc.com/2023/03/10/85-year-harvard-happiness-study-found-the-biggest-downside-of-retirement-that-no-one-talks-about.html.

Shemmassian, Shirag. 2023. "How Many Medical Schools Should I Apply to? Which Ones?" Shemmassian Academic Consulting. March 29, 2023. https://www.shemmassianconsulting.com/blog/how-many-medical-schools-should-i-apply-to.

Starecheski, Laura. 2015. "Take the ACE Quiz—and Learn What It Does and Doesn't Mean." NPR.Com. NPR. March 2, 2015. https://www.npr.org/sections/health-shots/2015/03/02/387007941/take-the-ace-quiz-and-learn-what-it-does-and-doesnt-mean.

"Strong Relationships, Strong Health." 2017. Better Health Channel. Victoria Department of Health & Human Services. October 2, 2017. https://www.betterhealth.vic.gov.au/health/healthyliving/Strong-relationships-strong-health.

"Summary of Hours of Service Regulations." 2022. FMCSA. US Department of Transportation. March 28, 2022. https://www.fmcsa.dot.gov/regulations/hours-service/summary-hours-service-regulations.

Talbot, Simon G., and Wendy Dean. 2018. "Physicians Aren't 'burning out.' They're Suffering from Moral Injury." STATNews. STAT. July 26, 2018. https://www.statnews.com/2018/07/26/physicians-not-burning-out-they-are-suffering-moral-injury/.

Tenny, Shane. 2020. "Here's Why Doctors Are Financially Depressed." KevinMD.Com. MedPage Today. March 5, 2020. https://www.kevinmd.com/2020/03/heres-why-doctors-are-financially-depressed.html.

Terlizzi, Emily P., and Benjamin Zablotsky. 2020. "Mental Health Treatment Among Adults: United States, 2019." National Center for Health Statistics. Centers for Disease Control and Prevention. September 23, 2020. https://www.cdc.gov/nchs/products/databriefs/db380.htm.

Thome, Janine, Maria Densmore, Georgia Koppe, Braeden Terpou, Jean Théberge, Margaret C. McKinnon, and Ruth A. Lanius. 2019. "Back to the Basics: Resting State Functional Connectivity of the Reticular Activation System in PTSD and Its Dissociative Subtype." *Chronic Stress* 3: 1–14. https://doi.org/10.1177/2470547019873663.

Thompson, Derek. 2019. "Workism Is Making Americans Miserable." *The Atlantic.* Atlantic Media Company. February 24, 2019. https://www.theatlantic.com/ideas/archive/2019/02/religion-workism-making-americans-miserable/583441/.

Townsley, Alexandra, and Rajani Katta. 2023. "Breaking the Stigma: Why Doctors Are Afraid to Seek Mental Health Treatment." KevinMD.Com. MedPage Today. February 13, 2023. https://www.kevinmd.com/2023/02/breaking-the-stigma-why-doctors-are-afraid-to-seek-mental-health-treatment.html.

Turner, Jimmy. 2022. "Physician, Know Thyself: A Self-Identity Crisis—The Physician Philosopher." *The Physician Philosopher*. March 3, 2022. https://thephysicianphilosopher.com/physician-know-thyself/.

Twain, Mark. 2005. *Pudd'nhead Wilson*. New York, NY: Bantam Classic.

Tyagi, Aditya. 2021. "'I Wasn't a Star Anymore': Miley Cyrus on Facing 'Identity Crisis' after 'Hannah Montana.'" *Republic World*. March 7, 2021. https://www.republicworld.com/entertainment-news/hollywood-news/i-wasnt-a-star-anymore-miley-cyrus-on-facing-identity-crisis-after-hannah-montana.html.

"US Average Hourly Earnings (I:USAHE)." 2023. YCharts. 2023. https://ycharts.com/indicators/us_average_hourly_earnings.

Vartabedian, Bryan. 2018. "Three A's of Physician Success: Availability, Affability, Ability." 33 Charts. March 30, 2018. https://33charts.com/availability-affability-ability/.

Wallace, Claire. 2023. "Physician suicide rate higher than any other profession." Becker's ASC Review. March 17, 2023. https://www.beckersasc.com/asc-news/physician-suicide-rate-higher-than-any-other-profession.html.

Wenn. 2021. "Zendaya Struggled with Identity Crisis as Lockdown Kicked In." Hollywood.Com. January 12, 2021. https://www.hollywood.com/celebrities/zendaya-struggled-with-identity-crisis-as-lockdown-kicked-in-60809526.

"What Is EMDR?" 2020. EMDR. 2020. https://www.emdr.com/what-is-emdr/.

"What's a Good MCAT Score?" 2023. Kaplan Test Prep. April 26, 2023. https://www.kaptest.com/study/mcat/whats-a-good-mcat-score/.

World Health Organization. 2021. "Closing the Leadership Gap: Gender Equity and Leadership in the Global Health and Care Workforce." June 2021. https://www.who.int/publications/i/item/9789240025905

Zagorsky, Jay L. 2022. "You Could Still Go Bankrupt Even If You Win the $2 Billion Poweball Jackpot." Fortune.Com. Fortune Magazine. November 8, 2022. https://fortune.com/2022/11/08/powerball-lotery-winners-could-still-go-bankrupt/.